LILY BENNETT

Hashimoto's Protocol: The Revolutionary Strategies for Balancing Thyroid Health

Navigate your healing journey with precision tactics and holistic remedies

First edition

This book was professionally typeset on Reedsy.
Find out more at reedsy.com

Contents

Introduction

In a world saturated with medical information, it is crucial to discover a source that not only imparts knowledge but also instills confidence and provides direction. This book aims to provide guidance and support for individuals who have recently been diagnosed with Hashimoto's Thyroiditis or have been managing this condition for a long time. Hashimoto's is a complex syndrome that affects various aspects of life, requiring a thorough understanding and personalized management.

My journey into the world of Hashimoto's Thyroiditis started more than ten years ago. At that time, I was not a patient, but a practitioner who closely observed the significant effects this condition had on the lives of my patients. Through the years, as I listened to the stories shared in the privacy of my office, I came to realize that despite the wealth of information available, there was a noticeable absence of genuine comprehension and practical advice specifically designed to address the distinct obstacles encountered by individuals with Hashimoto's. This book is a result of a strong desire to address that void.

My aim is to not just provide information, but to help you revolutionize your life with Hashimoto's. It's all about transforming knowledge into empowerment—the ability to take control of your health, make well-informed choices, and live a life that isn't dictated by your condition.

Throughout this book, you will explore the complex details of Hashimoto's Thyroiditis. Gain a solid understanding of Hashimoto's, an autoimmune disorder that causes the immune system to attack the thyroid gland, this leads to chronic inflammation and a variety of complex symptoms. You will delve into the important roles of the thyroid gland, an organ that plays a critical part in regulating metabolism, energy levels, and hormonal equilibrium.

Gaining knowledge is the initial stride towards empowerment. With this knowledge, we will explore the identification of the initial indications and symptoms of Hashimoto's. Being aware of the various symptoms, such as fatigue, weight changes, hair loss, and mood fluctuations, can be instrumental in recognizing when to seek the necessary assistance. Diagnosis can be a challenging process, often filled with uncertainty and mistakes. By familiarizing yourself with the different diagnostic tests and understanding their potential implications, you will be better equipped to navigate discussions with healthcare professionals and gain clarity on the process.

However, grasping the concept and identifying the issue is just the starting point. This book dives into the 'Hashimoto's Protocol', providing a thorough examination of various medical treatments, holistic practices, and dietary approaches. Learn about the various medications and therapies available to manage the disorder, as well as how integrative methods can work alongside them to offer relief and improve overall health.

Proper nutrition is essential for effectively managing chronic conditions, including Hashimoto's. Discover comprehensive advice on optimizing your body's nutrition to promote thyroid well-being and effectively address symptoms. This includes not only foods that nourish and heal but also those that might worsen your condition. With practical advice, meal plans, and recipes, you'll find it easier to make these dietary changes achievable and sustainable.

However, effectively managing Hashimoto's requires more than just focusing on diet and medication. Making changes to your lifestyle is essential for your overall health and happiness. This book offers practical advice on incorporating changes into your daily routine, including exercise routines that are safe and beneficial for individuals with Hashimoto's, as well as stress management techniques that can have a profound impact on your overall well-being. Quality sleep and how to achieve it will be a key focus, equipping you with the necessary tools to address one of the most prevalent challenges in thyroid disorders.

As you progress through the book, you will discover the most up-to-date treatments and the latest research that brings new hope to those affected. Exploring the connection between gut health and the immune system can provide valuable insights into managing Hashimoto's and enhancing your overall quality of life.

Lastly, living with Hashimoto's is more than just managing a chronic condition; it's about thriving despite it. Exploring coping mechanisms, establishing strong support systems, and providing access to resources for ongoing support and learning will be discussed, ensuring you have a network to rely on throughout your journey.

This book offers comprehensive guidance and support for individuals living with Hashimoto's Thyroiditis, ensuring that you have a trusted companion to help you navigate the complexities of this condition. Whether you are seeking validation, understanding, or fresh strategies to manage your condition, you will discover a comprehensive, empathetic, and practical approach here. I respect the challenges you face and provide you with the necessary tools to overcome them.

Welcome to an enlightening journey of understanding, wellness, and empowerment. Alright, let's get started.

1

Defining Hashimoto's Thyroiditis

"The thyroid is the engine of the body's train—small yet vital, often forgotten until it sputters and slows, disrupting the entire system."

Hashimoto's Thyroiditis is more than just a disorder; it's a complex interplay of the immune system, genetics, hormones, and environmental factors, all converging on one small but mighty gland in your neck. For many, the journey begins with subtle, seemingly disconnected symptoms: fatigue, weight gain, or even a sense of mental fog. These signs, often dismissed or misattributed, are the early whispers of a condition that will eventually affect every aspect of one's health.

Understanding Hashimoto's requires us to look deeper into the thyroid's role in our body's functions, beyond the surface-level symptoms and straightforward blood tests. This chapter sets the stage for a comprehensive exploration of Hashimoto's Thyroiditis, beginning with a clear definition of the disorder, its effects on the thyroid gland, and the common triggers and causes that lead to its development.

We'll uncover how this condition sneaks into the lives of those who carry it, often lying dormant until the right—or rather, the wrong—circumstances align. By the end of this chapter, you'll have a foundational understanding of Hashimoto's, equipping you with the knowledge necessary to navigate the complexities of this autoimmune disorder.

1.1. Defining Hashimoto's Thyroiditis

Hashimoto's Thyroiditis, commonly known as Hashimoto's, is more than just a condition. It takes us on an exploration of the intricate workings of the human immune system and its relationship with the thyroid, an organ that is often overlooked but plays a vital role in our overall health. This autoimmune disorder directs its attention toward the thyroid gland, leading to persistent inflammation and a range of metabolic disruptions. Understanding Hashimoto's requires a deep dive into the intricacies of how and why the immune system inexplicably turns against it.

The Immune System's Misguided Attack

Hashimoto's Thyroiditis is primarily caused by an immune system dysfunction. The body's defense mechanism constantly surveys for and eliminates harmful pathogens such as bacteria and viruses. Nevertheless, in Hashimoto's, the immune system fails to acknowledge the thyroid gland's cells as belonging to the body, instead targeting them as if they were any external threat. This attack is not an abrupt invasion but a slow, sneaky process that often goes unnoticed until noticeable symptoms appear.

Antibodies play a crucial role in the immune response by targeting the thyroid peroxidase (TPO) and thyroglobulin, which are essential enzymes in the production of thyroid hormones. With repeated assaults, the thyroid cells are gradually destroyed, causing a disruption in hormone production and resulting in a range of metabolic issues.

The Hormonal Havoc

When thyroid cells become damaged, the gland faces difficulties in producing sufficient thyroid hormone, resulting in hypothyroidism, which is the clinical term used to describe an underactive thyroid. This hormonal deficiency affects various systems throughout the body. Thyroid hormones, such as thyroxine (T4) and triiodothyronine (T3), have a significant impact on metabolism. They affect various aspects of the body, including energy levels, body temperature, and weight control.

Individuals with Hashimoto's disease commonly experience symptoms such as fatigue, weight gain, sensitivity to cold, and depression due to the decrease in hormone production. These signs indicate more than just a thyroid slowdown; they suggest that the body is facing challenges in maintaining its balance.

The Diagnostic Dilemma

Understanding the progression of Hashimoto's can be quite challenging. Some people may have the antibodies linked to the disorder without showing obvious symptoms, which can result in cases that go unnoticed or are wrongly diagnosed. By the time symptoms become severe enough to warrant medical investigation, the thyroid may have already sustained significant damage due to the disorder's insidious nature.

Diagnosis usually requires the identification of increased levels of thyroid antibodies in the bloodstream. Nevertheless, the mere presence of antibodies is insufficient to establish the presence of Hashimoto's disease. It is the combination of these antibodies and the presence of hypothyroid symptoms that usually leads to a conclusive diagnosis. Understanding and defining Hashimoto's can be quite a complex process, given the subtle dance of signs and markers involved.

Hashimoto's can have a wide range of presentations and pro-gressions. Some people may have a mild form of the disease with only a few noticeable symptoms, which can be managed with minimal intervention. For some individuals, the decrease in thyroid function can be quite severe, necessitating substantial changes to their lifestyle and the need for medical intervention. This variability introduces an additional level of complexity in determining the individual manifestations of Hashimoto's.

The disease can also have fluctuations, with periods of stability interrupted by episodes of worsening symptoms, commonly referred to as flare-ups. These fluctuations can be influenced by a range of factors, such as stress, infection, and other hormonal changes, which can make the clinical picture and management of Hashimoto's more complex.

Although the main focus of Hashimoto's is on the thyroid gland, it can have widespread effects throughout the body. It is worth noting that the disorder can coincide with other autoimmune diseases, like rheumatoid arthritis and type 1 diabetes, suggesting a wider autoimmune dysregulation. Patients with Hashimoto's often experience a variety of symptoms that can impact different systems in the body, ranging from gastrointestinal issues to reproductive abnormalities.

To truly comprehend Hashimoto's Thyroiditis, one must go beyond simply acknowledging its symptoms or relying on blood tests for diagnosis. Understanding the autoimmune nature of the disorder, the hormonal roles of the thyroid, and the systemic impact they have is crucial. Hashimoto's is a condition that goes beyond being just a thyroid disorder. It has a long-lasting impact on an individual's overall health and well-being.

Through this exploration, it becomes evident that understanding Hashimoto's Thyroiditis involves not only grasping the medical aspects but also acknowledging the personal experiences of those affected by the condition. As we explore the various aspects of Hashimoto's, we not only uncover the biological foundations but also the personal stories intertwined within the clinical narrative. This all-encompassing approach not only educates individuals, but also empowers them, equipping them with the necessary knowledge and tools to confidently navigate their condition.

1.2. The Role of the Thyroid in Body Functions

Nestled at the front of your neck, beneath a gentle contour of skin and the protective barrier of your Adam's apple, resides a vital yet often overlooked organ: the thyroid gland. This small but powerful gland, shaped like a butterfly, plays a crucial role in the intricate network of your body's functions. Gaining knowledge about the thyroid is important for individuals with Hashimoto's Thyroiditis, as well as for those fascinated by the intricate workings of human biology.

A Master Regulator in Disguise

The thyroid, although small in size, has a significant impact on the entire human body. It releases hormones that help control metabolism, which is the body's way of converting food and beverages into energy. This energy is not just the type that gets you out of bed in the morning or fuels your jog around the block; it is the essential energy that drives every cell in your body, from your brain cells contemplating the enigmas of the universe to the muscle cells facilitating your heart's rhythmic beat.

In this fascinating endocrine drama, the spotlight is on two key hormones: thyroxine (T4) and triiodothyronine (T3). The thyroid gland produces these hormones in response to thyroid-stimulating hormone (TSH), which is released by the pituitary gland in the brain. The delicate dance between TSH and thyroid hormones is a meticulously choreographed performance, executed with utmost precision to uphold metabolic equilibrium.

- Metabolic Maestro: Thyroid hormones play a key role in regulating your metabolism and affecting calorie burning and heart rate. These hormones have a significant impact on various bodily functions, ranging from digestion to regulating body temperature.

- Growth and Development Conductor: In children, thyroid hormones play a vital role in ensuring normal growth and development, especially for the brain. This role highlights the gland's significance from early life, extending its impact well beyond just metabolism.

- The Mood Modulator: The thyroid also plays a crucial role in regulating mood, although this is not widely recognized. Imbalances in thyroid hormone levels can cause noticeable changes in mood, highlighting the gland's influence on areas commonly associated with the brain.

Exploring Advanced Metabolic Processes

However, the thyroid's role also extends into more nuanced terrains:

- Thyroid hormones directly affect the heart and blood vessels, acting as a cardiovascular catalyst. They play a crucial role in maintaining a steady heart rate and ensuring efficient blood circulation throughout the body. This role emphasizes the importance of the thyroid in cardiovascular health.

- Thyroid hormones help maintain bone density by influencing the turnover of bone material. An imbalance can result in weakened bones that are more susceptible to fractures.

- Connections with Other Hormonal Pathways: The thyroid has connections with other hormonal systems, including the insulin-driven pathways involved in glucose metabolism and the adrenal glands' production of cortisol, which plays a role in managing stress and promoting body repair.

1 diabetes, your chances of developing the disease are much higher. There is evidence to suggest that certain genetic markers may increase an individual's vulnerability to autoimmune disorders, such as Hashimoto's.

Nevertheless, possessing a genetic predisposition does not necessarily mean that Hashimoto's will manifest in your case. Instead, it prepares the ground, leaving you more susceptible to other triggers that can kickstart the autoimmune response. Understanding why certain individuals develop the disease while others, despite similar genetic risks, do not, requires a deep understanding of the complex interplay between genetics and environmental factors.

Environmental Factors: The Unseen Threats

Environmental factors can play a significant role in influencing the development of Hashimoto's in individuals with a genetic predisposition. These factors can range from exposure to toxins to viral infections. For example, there is a connection between certain viruses such as Epstein-Barr and the development of autoimmune diseases. It is believed that these infections may potentially cause an exaggerated response from the immune system, resulting in a series of events where the immune system mistakenly targets the thyroid gland.

Environmental toxins, including heavy metals and specific chemicals, may also contribute to the issue. Exposure to substances such as mercury, commonly found in seafood or old dental fillings, along with other environmental pollutants, may potentially contribute to the development of autoimmune responses. These toxins have the potential to disrupt the immune system, which may result in immune dysregulation similar to that observed in Hashimoto's.

The Importance of Hormonal Changes

Hormonal fluctuations can be a significant trigger for Hashimoto's, especially in women. Hashimoto's Thyroiditis has a higher prevalence among women, and it tends to develop during times of hormonal changes, like pregnancy, menopause, or the regular menstrual cycle. During these times, the immune system is undergoing changes, which may potentially heighten the risk of developing autoimmune responses.

Pregnancy is a well-known trigger. Throughout pregnancy, the immune system of a woman is naturally suppressed to safe-guard the fetus from any potential harm. However, following childbirth, the immune system becomes more active again, occasionally in a forceful manner. This rebound effect has the potential to activate autoimmune diseases such as Hashimoto's. The hormonal changes that occur during menopause can also serve as a trigger, which could potentially explain the high number of women who are diagnosed with Hashimoto's during this period.

The Effects of Long-Term Stress

Stress is commonly referred to as the silent killer and has a significant impact on the development and advancement of autoimmune diseases, such as Hashimoto's. Chronic stress has the potential to disturb the delicate equilibrium of the immune system, resulting in an increased inflammatory response. This ongoing inflammation can eventually result in the immune system targeting the thyroid gland.

Stress can have an impact on the adrenal glands, which play a crucial role in producing cortisol, the body's main stress hormone. When the body experiences ongoing stress, it can disrupt the balance of cortisol levels, leading to potential impacts on thyroid function. The relationship between the adrenal glands and the thyroid is intricate, but it is evident that chronic stress can greatly influence the development of Hashimoto's disease, especially when combined with other factors such as genetic predisposition or environmental exposures.

Dietary Influences and Gut Health

Recent studies have shed light on the critical connection between diet and gut health in the development of autoimmune diseases. The gut houses a wide variety of bacteria that have important roles in digestion, immune function, and overall health. Nevertheless, if the gut's delicate equilibrium is disturbed - whether due to an unhealthy diet, the use of antibiotics, or ongoing stress – it can result in a condition referred to as "leaky gut."

An impaired intestinal barrier allows undigested food particles, toxins, and bacteria to permeate the gut lining and enter the bloodstream. This elicits an immune response, as the body perceives these substances as foreign intruders. Over time, the increased immune activity can result in autoimmune conditions such as Hashimoto's, where the immune system starts targeting the thyroid.

Some foods, especially those with gluten, have been found to possibly trigger Hashimoto's. Gluten has the potential to trigger an immune response in certain individuals, resulting in inflammation and, in more severe instances, the onset of autoimmune disorders. Many individuals with Hashimoto's have reported a reduction in symptoms and inflammation by eliminating gluten from their diet, although the exact connection between gluten and Hashimoto's is still under investigation.

The Cumulative Effect: A Perfect Storm

It's crucial to grasp that Hashimoto's Thyroiditis typically doesn't stem from a solitary cause. Instead, it's the combination of various factors – genetic, environmental, hormonal, and lifestyle – that contribute to the perfect storm. For instance, a woman who has a genetic predisposition to autoimmune diseases may not develop Hashimoto's until she goes through a period of significant stress, experiences hormonal changes during pregnancy, and gets exposed to a viral infection. This combination of triggers frequently contributes to the development of the disease.

By gaining knowledge about these common triggers and causes, individuals can take proactive steps to effectively manage their risk of developing Hashimoto's. One approach is to minimize exposure to environmental toxins, practice mindfulness to cope with stress, follow a nutritious diet, and closely monitor hormonal fluctuations, especially during critical periods such as pregnancy and menopause. With a deep understanding of the various factors that can trigger Hashimoto's, individuals can effectively navigate their health and potentially avoid the development or effectively manage the progression of the disease.

Conclusion

In this chapter, we've laid the groundwork for understanding Hashimoto's Thyroiditis, beginning with a definition of the condition that underscores its autoimmune nature and its profound impact on the thyroid gland. We've explored the thyroid's crucial role in regulating the body's functions, highlighting how disruptions to this small gland can lead to wide-reaching effects on metabolism, mood, and overall health.

Furthermore, we delved into the common triggers and causes of Hashimoto's, illustrating how a confluence of genetic predisposition, environmental factors, hormonal changes, stress, and diet can lead to the onset of this condition. Understanding these triggers not only provides insight into the origins of Hashimoto's but also offers pathways for managing and potentially mitigating its impact.

As we move forward in this book, this foundational knowledge will serve as a touchstone, guiding us through more detailed discussions on diagnosis, treatment, and lifestyle management. The complexities of Hashimoto's require a comprehensive approach, one that begins with a deep understanding of what this condition is and how it manifests. With this knowledge in hand, you are better equipped to confront and manage Hashimoto's Thyroiditis with informed confidence.

2

Diagnosis and Early Signs

"It's not the disease itself that changes a life; it's the delay in diagnosing it."

Hashimoto's Thyroiditis is often called the "great masquerader" due to its wide range of symptoms that can easily be mistaken for other conditions. Fatigue, weight gain, mood swings—these signs can seem innocuous or be attributed to stress, aging, or lifestyle. However, behind these symptoms lies a more complex story of an autoimmune attack on the thyroid gland, gradually undermining its ability to function. This chapter explores the critical steps of recognizing the early signs of Hashimoto's and the importance of timely diagnosis.

Understanding the symptoms and their subtle cues is only the beginning. The path to diagnosis often involves a series of diagnostic tests that not only confirm the presence of the disease but also help gauge its progression. Early detection is key to managing Hashimoto's effectively and preventing long-term complications. As you navigate through this chapter, you'll discover how to recognize the red flags, understand diagnostic tests, and appreciate the profound importance of catching Hashimoto's in its earliest stages.

2.1. Recognizing the Symptoms

Hashimoto's Thyroiditis is commonly referred to as a "silent" disease, not because it lacks symptoms, but due to the subtle and varied nature of its symptoms, which can often be mistaken for other conditions. Recognizing these symptoms is an important initial step toward a diagnosis that can have a significant impact on one's overall health. However, this process is far from being simple. Hashimoto's can manifest in various ways, with symptoms that fluctuate, often resulting in a diagnosis that is delayed. Having a good grasp of these symptoms, including both the typical ones and the more subtle ones, can give individuals the confidence to seek the necessary medical care early on, preventing the disease from advancing further.

The Silent Beginning

Recognizing Hashimoto's Thyroiditis can be challenging due to its subtle and gradual onset. Unlike certain conditions that manifest themselves abruptly and dramatically, Hashimoto tends to gradually develop over time. The gradual nature of this progression often leads to the initial symptoms being easily dismissed or misattributed to factors like stress, aging, or lifestyle choices.

Fatigue is a frequently reported symptom, but unfortunately, it is often overlooked. We all go through periods of fatigue occasionally, and it's easy to dismiss ongoing tiredness as a consequence of a hectic schedule, inadequate sleep, or insufficient physical activity. However, the fatigue linked to Hashimoto's is a profound and persistent exhaustion that does not alleviate even with rest. It's the type of fatigue that makes getting out of bed in the morning seem like an impossible feat, that persists even after a restful night's sleep, and that can permeate every aspect of your life, impacting your work, relationships, and overall state of mind.

The Physical Manifestations

As Hashimoto's advances, the thyroid gland's hormone production decreases, resulting in a range of physical symptoms. Weight gain can be a common early sign, often accompanied by a frustrating inability to shed pounds despite dedicated diet and exercise. This weight gain may not be particularly significant, but it can be quite persistent and frustrating, as it appears to go against the typical principles of calorie intake and expenditure.

Another common symptom is feeling cold easily. Individuals with Hashimoto's disease frequently feel the need to grab a sweater or blanket when others around them are perfectly comfortable. One possible reason for feeling more sensitive to cold is the decrease in thyroid hormone levels, which can slow down metabolism and impact the body's ability to produce and retain heat.

Skin and hair changes are commonly observed. Changes in the skin's texture and hair quality are common symptoms that can occur. Thinning of the eyebrows, especially the outer third, is often observed in individuals with hypothyroidism. These changes, although not posing any immediate danger, can greatly affect a person's self-confidence and overall well-being.

Digestive issues are frequently encountered but often go unnoticed. Chronic constipation is a common issue for individuals with Hashimoto's, as the reduced metabolism can impact the movement of the digestive tract. On the other hand, certain people may encounter bloating, indigestion, or even unexplained nausea.

The Emotional and Cognitive Impact

Hashimoto's can have an impact on both the physical and mental well-being. Depression and anxiety often affect individuals with the condition, and these symptoms can be quite distressing as they tend to manifest before the more well-known physical symptoms. It's quite common for individuals with undiagnosed Hashimoto's to undergo years of treatment for depression or anxiety before the root cause, the underlying thyroid issue, is finally recognized.

Brain fog is a cognitive symptom that can have a significant impact on one's daily life. Individuals with Hashimoto's frequently express a sense of cognitive sluggishness or a foggy state that hampers their ability to focus, recall information, or maintain mental clarity. It can have an impact on various aspects of life, ranging from work productivity to basic activities such as recalling a shopping list or engaging in a conversation.

It is important to recognize these emotional and cognitive symptoms as they are often mistakenly attributed to other causes. One might mistakenly attribute these symptoms to the natural aging process, stress, or a difficult period, when in reality, they could be indicative of thyroid dysfunction.

The Fluctuating Symptoms

It is quite perplexing how the symptoms of Hashimoto's can vary over time. There might be times when symptoms worsen, referred to as flare-ups, followed by periods of improvement, which can give a false sense of recovery. This fluctuation can pose a challenge for individuals and their doctors in identifying the disease's pattern.

When flare-ups occur, symptoms such as fatigue, joint pain, and mood swings can become more intense, making it difficult to navigate daily life. Flare-ups can be triggered by different factors such as stress, illness, or hormonal changes, and adjustments in management strategies are often necessary.

It is crucial to pay attention to your body and make note of any persistent or unusual changes, considering the broad spectrum of symptoms linked to Hashimoto's. Keeping a symptom journal can be an incredibly useful resource. By consistently documenting your symptoms on a regular basis, you can uncover patterns that may have otherwise escaped your attention. This record can also serve as a valuable resource when discussing your concerns with your healthcare provider, enabling them to gain a comprehensive understanding and potentially consider Hashimoto's as a potential diagnosis.

It's important to assert yourself if you have concerns about your health. Given the similarity of symptoms, it is not uncommon for individuals to receive a misdiagnosis or be informed that their symptoms are a result of stress or aging. If you believe your symptoms are being disregarded, it may be beneficial to consider seeking a second opinion or asking for a referral to a specialist who focuses on thyroid disorders, such as an endocrinologist.

Understanding the symptoms of Hashimoto's Thyroiditis is key in order to receive the correct diagnosis and treatment. Being mindful of your physical well-being and staying attuned to any shifts in your body can be crucial, as symptoms can often be diverse and elusive. In the following section, we will explore the diagnostic process, including the various tests and evaluations that can help determine if Hashimoto's is the underlying cause of your symptoms. Recognizing these indicators and taking proactive steps is critical for gaining control over your well-being and embarking on the path to effectively managing this condition.

2.2. Diagnostic Tests and Interpretation

In dealing with Hashimoto's Thyroiditis, finding the right diagnosis can sometimes feel like solving a complex puzzle. The symptoms can present in a wide range, with subtle manifestations that may resemble those of numerous other conditions. Diagnostic tests play a crucial role in confirming the presence of Hashimoto's and gaining a comprehensive understanding of its impact on the thyroid gland. These tests provide valuable insights into the body's internal processes, offering essential information that helps with both diagnosis and treatment. However, properly interpreting these tests goes beyond simply examining the numerical values; it necessitates a comprehensive understanding of the significance of each result and its relevance to overall thyroid well-being.

The Importance of Blood Tests in Diagnosis

Diagnosing Hashimoto's Thyroiditis relies heavily on blood tests that assess the levels of thyroid hormones and thyroid antibodies. These tests provide valuable insights into thyroid function and immune activity, allowing us to determine if the thyroid is functioning properly and if the immune system is specifically targeting the thyroid.

Thyroid-Stimulating Hormone (TSH): When there is a suspicion of thyroid dysfunction, one of the initial tests usually requested is the measurement of Thyroid-Stimulating Hormone (TSH). TSH is produced by the pituitary gland and serves as a signal to the thyroid, directing it to produce thyroid hormones. When it comes to Hashimoto's, a high TSH level is often a sign that the thyroid isn't producing sufficient hormones. As a result, the pituitary gland increases its production of TSH in an effort to stimulate the thyroid. Nevertheless, an elevated TSH alone does not provide confirmation of Hashimoto's; it merely suggests that the thyroid might not be functioning correctly.

Free Thyroxine (Free T4): Free T4 levels are measured in

addition to TSH. Free T4 is a key hormone that is synthesized by the thyroid gland. It is considered "free" as it is not bound to proteins in the blood, making it readily available for the body to utilize. In cases of Hashimoto's disease, the Free T4 level can be lower, indicating a decrease in the thyroid's ability to produce this hormone. Having a low Free T4 and an elevated TSH is a strong indication of hypothyroidism, but it does not definitively identify Hashimoto's as the underlying cause.

Thyroid Peroxidase Antibodies (TPOAb) are an important factor to consider. Thyroid antibodies are tested to specifically diagnose Hashimoto's. Thyroid Peroxidase Antibodies (TPOAb) are frequently elevated in cases of Hashimoto's disease. These antibodies specifically target thyroid peroxidase, which is a key enzyme involved in the production of thyroid hormones. High TPOAb levels are a clear indication that the immune system is targeting the thyroid, which strongly suggests the presence of Hashimoto's Thyroiditis.

Thyroglobulin Antibodies (TgAb): Another antibody that could be considered for testing is Thyroglobulin Antibodies (TgAb). Thyroglobulin is a protein that is produced by the thyroid gland. In certain instances of Hashimoto's, the immune system generates antibodies against it. Although TgAb is not as frequently elevated as TPOAb, it can still be helpful in confirming a diagnosis of Hashimoto's, particularly when TPOAb levels are not elevated.

Interpreting the Results

Deciphering these blood test results can be quite complex. Having a deep understanding of the complex interactions between different hormones and antibodies, along with careful consideration of the patient's symptoms and medical history, is critical.

Gaining Insight into TSH and T4 Levels: Having elevated TSH and low Free T4 levels usually point towards hypothyroidism, although they do not definitively establish Hashimoto's as the cause. Thyroid antibodies play a crucial role in distinguishing Hashimoto's from other forms of thyroid dysfunction, as hypothyroidism can have various causes. When TSH levels are high but Free T4 levels remain within the normal range, it is commonly known as subclinical hypothyroidism. At this early stage of thyroid dysfunction, it is important to keep an eye on the situation and, in certain instances, consider treatment. This is particularly true if there are thyroid antibodies present, which could indicate Hashimoto's.

The Importance of Antibody Levels: Having thyroid antibodies, especially TPOAb, is a reliable sign of Hashimoto's Thyroiditis. It is worth mentioning that the level of antibodies does not always indicate the severity of the disease. It is interesting to note that individuals can exhibit varying degrees of symptoms, regardless of their antibody levels. Some may experience mild or even no symptoms, despite having high antibody levels, while others with lower antibody levels may suffer from more severe disease. This variability highlights the significance of considering the entire clinical picture, rather than focusing solely on individual test results.

Beyond the Blood Tests

Although blood tests are crucial for diagnosing Hashimoto, there are other diagnostic tools that can be used as well. Additional diagnostic tests may sometimes be necessary to obtain a more comprehensive understanding of thyroid health and to eliminate the possibility of other conditions.

Ultrasound Imaging

An ultrasound of the thyroid can provide important insights into the size, shape, and structure of the gland. The thyroid in Hashimoto's disease frequently exhibits irregularities, such as inflammation or atrophy. Small growths known as nodules may also be present. When nodules are present alongside other signs of Hashimoto's, it can provide additional support for the diagnosis, as they are often common and benign.

Fine-Needle Aspiration (FNA)

If nodules are detected, a fine-needle aspiration (FNA) biopsy may be performed. This procedure requires the use of a fine needle to extract a small tissue sample from the nodule, which is subsequently examined under a microscope. FNA is commonly utilized to assess nodules for cancer. However, it can also offer insights into the presence of lymphocytes and other immune cells that are indicative of Hashimoto's.

Diagnostic tests are extremely useful, but they don't provide a complete picture. Tracking symptoms over time can be essential in the diagnostic process, as Hashimoto's symptoms can fluctuate and differ significantly from person to person. Maintaining a comprehensive log of symptoms, including their timing, intensity, and possible triggers, can offer your healthcare provider valuable insights for analyzing test results and reaching a diagnosis.

The Art of Diagnosis

Diagnosing Hashimoto's Thyroiditis requires a combination of expertise and precision. It requires assembling the pieces of the puzzle, including symptoms, blood tests, imaging studies, and occasionally biopsies, to reach a diagnosis. It's a complex procedure that necessitates a thorough comprehension of the thyroid and immune system, as well as attentive listening and thoughtful consideration of the patient's perspective.

For patients, the journey toward a diagnosis can be incredibly frustrating, particularly when symptoms are ambiguous or disregarded as mere consequences of stress or the natural aging process. It is crucial to prioritize comprehensive testing and consider seeking a second opinion when needed to guarantee an accurate diagnosis.

Once a diagnosis of Hashimoto's is established, it provides a variety of management and treatment options that are customized to meet the individual's specific needs. Having a clear understanding of the results of diagnostic tests and their correlation with your symptoms is key at the beginning of this journey. With this knowledge in hand, you and your healthcare provider can collaborate to create a customized plan to effectively manage Hashimoto's and enhance your thyroid health. Throughout this book, we will delve deeper into these management strategies, providing you with the knowledge and guidance to confidently navigate the complexities of Hashimoto's.

2.3. The Importance of Early Detection

Early detection is a key concept in the medical field, especially when it comes to Hashimoto's Thyroiditis. Identifying Hashimoto early is crucial to prevent significant damage to the thyroid and the unraveling of the body's systems due to insufficient thyroid hormone production. Identifying the disease at an early stage enables prompt intervention, increasing the likelihood of effectively managing the condition, alleviating symptoms, and averting potential complications that could greatly affect one's overall well-being.

The Quiet Progression of Hashimoto's

Hashimoto's Thyroiditis is a condition that can progress without much notice, gradually affecting the thyroid gland's functionality. It is common for individuals to overlook the early signs of a thyroid disorder, such as fatigue, mild depression, and subtle weight gain, which can persist for months or even years. When more noticeable symptoms such as extreme exhaustion, substantial weight gain, and noticeable changes in mood become apparent, it is possible that the thyroid has already suffered significant damage.

Early detection plays a crucial role in this matter. Through early detection of the disease, when symptoms may still be subtle or barely noticeable, measures can be taken to slow down its advancement. Identifying Hashimoto's in its early stages enables a proactive approach to managing the disease and minimizing its impact on the body.

The Advantages of Early Intervention

Early detection offers a significant advantage by allowing for timely initiation of appropriate treatments, preventing substantial thyroid damage. Hashimoto's is a long-term condition where the immune system gradually destroys thyroid cells. Over time, the gradual destruction of the gland results in a decreased production of vital hormones, ultimately causing hypothyroidism. Early intervention can help in preserving thyroid function, potentially extending the time before hormone replacement therapy becomes necessary.

In addition, receiving treatment early can help relieve symptoms that may start off as mild but can worsen over time. Experiencing fatigue, mental fog, and mood disturbances can significantly impact one's quality of life, making it challenging to perform well at work, maintain healthy relationships, and participate in activities that were once pleasurable. Addressing these symptoms promptly can help prevent a significant decline in daily functioning and overall well-being.

Early detection also allows for the chance to educate and make lifestyle changes that can have a positive effect on the progression of the disease. Patients who receive an early diagnosis have the opportunity to gain knowledge about their condition and make proactive changes to promote their thyroid health. This can be achieved through dietary adjustments, stress management techniques, and other lifestyle modifications. By implementing these modifications at an early stage, individuals can frequently alleviate the severity of symptoms and enhance their long-term outlook.

Identifying the Risk Factors

Recognizing individuals who may be prone to developing Hashimoto's Thyroiditis is crucial for early detection. Having a good grasp of the risk factors can help patients and healthcare providers stay alert for any potential signs of the disease.

Individuals who have a family history of autoimmune diseases, especially thyroid disorders, have a higher likelihood of developing Hashimoto's. In the same way, women, particularly those in their middle age, have a higher likelihood of being impacted. By identifying these risk factors, it enables focused screening and monitoring, resulting in the potential for earlier detection and treatment.

In addition, it's important for individuals with other autoimmune conditions, such as type 1 diabetes or rheumatoid arthritis, to be aware of their heightened risk for Hashimoto's. Regular thyroid function tests for these patients can be instrumental in detecting the disease early on, enabling timely intervention. Recognizing the interconnections between autoimmune conditions underscores the significance of taking a holistic approach to managing chronic illnesses.

The Importance of Regular Screening

Regular screening for thyroid dysfunction is an essential component of early detection. Routine screening for individuals at high risk or those displaying symptoms suggestive of thyroid dysfunction can be vital for saving lives. Screening usually includes basic blood tests to assess TSH and thyroid hormone levels, along with tests for thyroid antibodies. These tests have the ability to identify thyroid problems before they show any symptoms, enabling timely intervention.

Regular monitoring is important for patients who have been

diagnosed with mild hypothyroidism or subclinical thyroid dysfunction. Monitoring thyroid function is important to identify when treatment may be needed, even if it's not necessary at the moment. It also offers a chance to modify treatment as necessary, guaranteeing the best possible management of the condition.

Untreated Hashimoto's can have extensive complications, impacting various systems in the body. If hypothyroidism is not treated, it can result in elevated cholesterol levels, heart disease, and in severe instances, myxedema coma, a critical condition that poses a risk to life. It can also worsen symptoms of depression and anxiety, affect fertility, and lead to complications during pregnancy.

By detecting Hashimoto's in its early stages and initiating treatment promptly, it is possible to prevent or reduce the risk of complications. Starting thyroid hormone replacement therapy early can be beneficial in maintaining healthy cholesterol levels and reducing the risk of heart disease. It is important to manage thyroid function before pregnancy in order to minimize the risk of complications for both the mother and baby.

In addition, detecting the condition early enables the development of treatment plans that are tailored to each individual's needs. With diligent monitoring of thyroid function and appropriate adjustments to treatment, healthcare providers can assist patients in achieving and maintaining optimal thyroid health. This proactive approach can help patients avoid the fluctuating symptoms often associated with inadequately controlled thyroid disease.

Empowering Patients Through Awareness

Early detection empowers patients and gives them a sense of control. Having a good understanding of the early signs and symptoms of Hashimoto's, the significance of regular screening, and the risk factors linked to the disease can empower patients to manage their health effectively. Early detection empowers patients to take a proactive approach to their healthcare, actively participating in their treatment and well-being.

This sense of empowerment goes beyond the individual patient. Spreading awareness and knowledge about the significance of early detection can create a ripple effect, motivating individuals, their loved ones, and communities to prioritize thyroid health. When individuals grasp the indicators to be mindful of and the significance of prompt intervention, they tend to promptly seek medical assistance, resulting in timely diagnosis and improved results.

Early detection is crucial in the battle against Hashimoto's Thyroiditis. With a keen eye for early indicators, a thorough grasp of the factors that increase susceptibility, and a commitment to consistent screening, we can detect the illness before it inflicts substantial harm on the body. Early intervention has a significant impact on health outcomes and greatly improves the quality of life for individuals, enabling them to live a vibrant and fulfilling life despite their diagnosis.

Conclusion

In this chapter, we've journeyed through the often murky waters of diagnosing Hashimoto's Thyroiditis, highlighting the importance of recognizing early symptoms that can easily be dismissed or overlooked. From the insidious onset of fatigue and weight gain to the more complex symptoms that affect mental clarity and mood, understanding these signs can set the stage for a timely diagnosis.

We've also delved into the critical role of diagnostic tests, explaining how each test contributes to the broader picture of thyroid health. Knowing what to look for in test results and interpreting them correctly can make all the difference in identifying Hashimoto's before significant damage occurs. Early detection isn't just about finding the disease; it's about preventing complications, improving treatment outcomes, and empowering individuals to take control of their health journey.

As we conclude this chapter, it's clear that early recognition and diagnosis are the cornerstones of effective Hashimoto's management. Armed with this knowledge, you are now better prepared to advocate for your health and pursue a path of proactive care, ensuring that Hashimoto's is managed with the foresight and understanding it demands. As we move forward, the focus will shift towards treatment options and lifestyle adjustments that can further enhance the quality of life for those living with this condition.

3

The Hashimoto's Protocol: A Strategic Overview

"Healing is not a one-size-fits-all endeavor; it's a personal journey shaped by understanding, patience, and the willingness to adapt."

Living with Hashimoto's Thyroiditis can feel like navigating a complex maze, where every twist and turn presents new challenges and uncertainties. The symptoms are varied, the triggers are numerous, and the path to wellness is far from linear. In such a landscape, finding a clear and effective strategy for managing the condition is essential. This is where the Hashimoto's Protocol comes in—a comprehensive, strategic approach designed to address the root causes of the disease, manage symptoms, and promote long-term health.

In this chapter, we'll dive deep into the principles that form the foundation of the Hashimoto's Protocol, exploring the essential components that make this approach both unique

40

and effective. From understanding the underlying triggers of Hashimoto's to implementing personalized dietary, lifestyle, and supplementation strategies, we'll uncover how this protocol empowers individuals to take control of their health. But more importantly, we'll emphasize the importance of tailoring this approach to meet individual needs, recognizing that each person's journey with Hashimoto's is as unique as their fingerprint. By the end of this chapter, you will be equipped with the knowledge and tools to begin crafting a personalized plan that aligns with your specific circumstances and health goals.

3.1. Principles of the Protocol

The experience of navigating Hashimoto's Thyroiditis is highly individual, yet it revolves around a common desire: the quest for equilibrium and good health. Successfully navigating this path necessitates a comprehensive approach that takes into account individual needs and focuses on addressing the root causes of the disease, effectively managing symptoms, and fostering overall well-being. The Hashimoto Protocol is founded on a deep appreciation for the individuality of each person, providing a well-structured approach to address the intricate challenges posed by this autoimmune condition. Understanding the root cause of the disease and taking a comprehensive, holistic approach is critical, going beyond just managing symptoms.

Gaining Insight into the Underlying Factors

Central to the Hashimoto's Protocol is a core principle: gaining a comprehensive understanding of the disease's underlying causes and taking steps to address them. This protocol goes beyond conventional treatments that often only address symptoms, delving into the underlying causes. Hashimoto's extends beyond a mere thyroid issue. It encompasses an autoimmune condition that affects the immune system, the gut, and a range of environmental and lifestyle factors. For effective management of Hashimoto's, it is crucial to first identify and address the underlying triggers.

I always begin with a comprehensive assessment to identify any potential factors that could be triggering the immune system's unwarranted assault on the thyroid. One possible approach is to evaluate for food sensitivities, chronic infections, toxin exposures, and other potential triggers. Through the identification of these underlying issues, the protocol strives to minimize the autoimmune response, thus safeguarding thyroid function and relieving symptoms.

Restoring Gut Health

Restoring gut health is a pivotal principle of the Hashimoto's Protocol. The gut is commonly known as the body's "second brain," and its well-being is closely linked to immune function. Many individuals with Hashimoto's experience compromised gut health, resulting in a condition called "leaky gut." This occurs when the lining of the gut becomes permeable, allowing undigested food particles, toxins, and microbes to enter the bloodstream. This can stimulate an immune response that may worsen autoimmune conditions, such as Hashimoto's.

The protocol prioritizes the healing of the gut as a crucial first step in managing Hashimoto's. It is important to follow a diet that promotes gut healing by focusing on anti-inflammatory and nutrient-dense foods. It also involves removing foods that can cause inflammation and affect gut health, like gluten, dairy, and processed foods. Through the restoration of gut integrity, the immune system can be effectively regulated, leading to a reduction in the autoimmune attack on the thyroid and an overall improvement in health.

Achieving Hormonal Balance

One important aspect of the Hashimoto's Protocol is maintaining a healthy balance of hormones. Hashimoto's has a wide-ranging impact on various hormones, including those related to the thyroid, adrenal glands, sex hormones, and even insulin regulation. The protocol acknowledges the intricate relationship between these hormonal systems and the significance of attaining equilibrium for overall well-being.

Dealing with hormonal balance requires taking steps to support the body's natural hormone production and ensuring that each hormone system is operating at its best. When it comes to the thyroid, it may involve the use of thyroid hormone replacement if necessary. Additionally, it encompasses promoting adrenal health by implementing stress management techniques, ensuring sufficient sleep, and maintaining a balanced diet. With the goal of promoting a harmonious internal environment and mitigating the effects of Hashimoto's on the body, the protocol provides comprehensive support for all hormonal systems, including thyroid function.

Reducing Inflammation

As an expert in the field of endocrinology, it is well-known that inflammation plays a significant role in autoimmune diseases, including Hashimoto's. Chronic inflammation not only worsens thyroid damage but also adds to the overall symptom burden faced by individuals with Hashimoto's. Reducing inflammation throughout the body is a fundamental principle of Hashimoto's Protocol.

Addressing inflammation requires a comprehensive strategy that encompasses adjustments to your diet, alterations to your lifestyle, and the incorporation of specific supplements. It is recommended to include anti-inflammatory foods in your diet, such as leafy greens, fatty fish, and berries. On the other hand, it is advisable to limit the consumption of inflammatory foods like refined sugars and trans fats. Incorporating stress reduction techniques such as meditation and yoga into the protocol is crucial. These practices aid in lowering cortisol levels and mitigating inflammatory responses. In addition, specific supplements like omega-3 fatty acids, turmeric, and antioxidants can offer focused support in reducing inflammation.

Supporting Detoxification

Detoxification is an essential principle of the Hashimoto's Protocol. In today's modern society, it is almost impossible to escape the presence of environmental toxins, which can greatly affect the health of the thyroid gland. Toxins such as heavy metals, pesticides, and endocrine disruptors can have a detrimental effect on thyroid function and play a role in the autoimmune response observed in Hashimoto's.

The protocol highlights the importance of aiding the body's inherent detoxification processes in order to eliminate these harmful substances and minimize their effects on the thyroid and immune system. It is important to focus on reducing exposure to toxins by adopting clean living practices. Additionally, one can improve the body's detoxification process by paying attention to nutrition, hydration, and incorporating targeted supplements such as milk thistle, which aids in supporting liver function. Engaging in regular physical activity and incorporating practices such as sauna therapy can effectively stimulate detoxification pathways. This, in turn, aids in the elimination of toxins through sweat and enhances lymphatic drainage.

Optimizing Nutrition and Lifestyle

A well-rounded, nourishing diet and a lifestyle that promotes good health are essential components of the Hashimoto's Protocol. This principle emphasizes the importance of not only avoiding foods that may cause inflammation or gut problems, but also making sure the body gets the necessary nutrients to promote thyroid health and overall well-being. For optimal thyroid function and a strong immune system, it is crucial to include nutrients like selenium, zinc, iodine, and vitamins D and B12 in your diet. The protocol emphasizes the consumption of foods that are abundant in these essential nutrients.

Aside from making changes to your diet, it's important to also incorporate lifestyle modifications into the protocol. Regular exercise, sufficient sleep, effective stress management, and mindfulness practices are all highlighted as essential elements of a healthy lifestyle that promotes optimal thyroid function. By implementing these strategies, individuals with Hashimoto's can improve their overall well-being, alleviate symptoms, and enjoy a better quality of life.

Personal Empowerment and Education

One of the key principles of Hashimoto's Protocol is the importance of empowering oneself through education. Managing Hashimoto's is a process that necessitates acquiring knowledge, comprehension, and a dedication to assuming responsibility for one's well-being. The protocol emphasizes the importance of individuals educating themselves about their condition, understanding each component of the protocol, and actively participating in their healthcare decisions.

This principle goes beyond simply adhering to a set of guidelines. It involves taking a proactive stance toward your health, comprehending the reasoning behind each recommendation, and being open to making necessary adjustments. Understanding your body's signals, identifying any issues, and finding the necessary resources and guidance to make well-informed decisions about your health are crucial.

With a focus on these fundamental principles, the Hashimoto's Protocol offers a thorough framework for effectively managing Hashimoto's Thyroiditis. It focuses on the underlying factors contributing to the disease, promotes holistic well-being, and encourages individuals to actively manage their health. Having a strong grasp of these principles, you are ready to start implementing the protocol and taking the necessary steps to effectively manage your Hashimoto's.

3.2. Tailoring the Approach to Individual Needs

Hashimoto's Thyroiditis varies in its impact on different individuals. Every individual's encounter with this autoimmune disorder can differ greatly, affected by various elements such as genetic makeup, lifestyle choices, environmental influences, and personal medical background. Due to the variability, it is rare for a one-size-fits-all approach to be effective. The Hashimoto's Protocol is designed to be versatile and accommodating, acknowledging that the optimal approach to healing and well-being is one that is customized to meet the unique requirements of each person. Understanding your body's unique needs and responding accordingly is key to this personalized approach. It goes beyond simply selecting supplements or making dietary changes. It's about recognizing the nuances of your own body.

Understanding Your Individual Requirements

Understanding your own health profile is crucial when customizing the Hashimoto's Protocol to meet your specific needs. Understanding your symptoms and examining lab reports are just the tip of the iceberg. It's crucial to take a comprehensive approach to your overall well-being. Reflect on your personal history: Have you ever gone through periods of intense stress? Have any members of your family experienced autoimmune diseases? Have you possibly encountered any environmental toxins throughout the years? All these factors are essential in determining your individual health profile and, consequently, how Hashimoto's disease presents itself in your body.

Consider your symptoms as well. Some individuals may experience fatigue and weight gain as symptoms of Hashimoto's, while others may have more severe digestive issues or mental fog. Understanding the combination and severity of symptoms can provide valuable insights into internal processes and areas that require additional attention. For example, if digestive issues are prominent, it may be more urgent to focus on improving gut health. If fatigue is the main concern, it may be important to prioritize supporting adrenal function.

Personalized Nutritional Strategies

Managing Hashimoto's requires making dietary adjustments, as what may be effective for one person may not be for another. Different people may benefit from different dietary approaches, such as gluten-free, dairy-free, or other nutritional changes. It's important to pay close attention to your body's signals and adjust your diet accordingly, depending on how your body reacts to different foods.

An effective strategy for determining your ideal diet involves trying an elimination diet. This method requires temporarily removing common inflammatory foods like gluten, dairy, soy, and sugar, and then slowly reintroducing them one by one. This process assists in determining which foods may be causing symptoms and which ones are easily tolerated. Maintain a thorough food journal during this period to monitor your symptoms and how your body reacts to various foods. By analyzing your body's response to different dietary changes, you can gain valuable insights and customize your nutrition plan accordingly.

In addition to removing troublesome foods, it is crucial to prioritize the inclusion of nutrient-rich choices that promote thyroid and overall well-being. It is highly recommended to include foods that are abundant in selenium, zinc, iodine, and antioxidants as regular components of your diet. It is important to customize your nutrition plan to suit your specific needs and tolerances, as the amounts and sources of nutrients can vary.

Targeted Supplementation

Supplements can be instrumental in promoting thyroid health and effectively managing Hashimoto's. However, it is key to customize supplementation to suit each individual's needs, just like with diet. It is wise to consult with a healthcare provider to assess your individual requirements before incorporating any supplements into your routine. Typically, a thorough analysis of blood work is conducted to detect any potential deficiencies or imbalances.

Supplementing these nutrients might be beneficial if your tests reveal low levels of vitamin D or B12. If you're dealing with high levels of inflammation, incorporating anti-inflammatory supplements such as omega-3 fatty acids or turmeric into your routine may prove beneficial. Certain individuals may find it beneficial to incorporate supplements that promote adrenal health, gut healing, or detoxification, depending on their specific needs and circumstances.

Keep in mind that excessive intake of supplements may not always be beneficial. Adopting a personalized approach that caters to your unique requirements, as opposed to a one-size-fits-all method involving various supplements, proves to be more efficient and secure in the long term. Consistent monitoring and adjustments, considering your response and changes in your condition, are crucial for effective supplementation.

Making Adjustments to Your Lifestyle

Personalizing lifestyle changes is important for effectively managing Hashimoto's. For certain individuals, stress management may be of utmost importance. Chronic stress has the potential to worsen autoimmune conditions as it can lead to increased inflammation and hormonal imbalances. If you discover that stress has a significant impact on your symptoms, incorporating regular stress-reducing practices like meditation, yoga, or deep breathing exercises can have a transformative effect.

Some individuals may benefit from placing greater emphasis on enhancing sleep quality or integrating regular physical activity into their routine. Regular physical activity is advantageous for maintaining good health and can contribute to the proper functioning of the thyroid gland. However, it is vital to strike a harmonious balance that suits your individual body. Excessive exercise may not yield the desired results, particularly if one is worried about adrenal fatigue, whereas insufficient physical activity can contribute to weight gain and reduced energy levels. Discovering the optimal form and intensity of physical activity that leaves you energized instead of exhausted is crucial for effectively managing Hashimoto's.

Customization is essential when it comes to sleep. People with Hashimoto's often have trouble sleeping, which can make their symptoms worse. Creating a customized sleep hygiene routine that incorporates a consistent sleep schedule, a calming bedtime routine, and a sleep-friendly environment can enhance the quality of sleep and, in turn, promote better overall health.

Collaborating with a Healthcare Team

Understanding the intricacies of Hashimoto's goes beyond mere trial and error. It calls for a collaborative effort with a healthcare team well-versed in autoimmune conditions. Seeking input from various healthcare professionals, such as an endocrinologist, nutritionist, and functional medicine practitioner, can offer a comprehensive viewpoint and assist in developing a personalized health plan.

Your healthcare team can assist in interpreting test results, offering guidance on dietary changes, suggesting targeted supplements, and providing support for implementing lifestyle modifications. Collaborating with your healthcare providers ensures that you're not going through this journey by yourself and that you have the necessary expertise and resources to effectively manage your condition.

Paying Attention to Your Body

Understanding your body's signals is crucial when customizing the Hashimoto's Protocol to suit your individual needs. Take note of your body's response to different foods, supplements, and activities. Your body frequently provides signals, ranging from subtle to more obvious, about its needs or any issues it may be experiencing.

Building body awareness requires dedication and effort, but it is essential for effectively managing Hashimoto's. By paying close attention to how your body reacts, you can make better choices regarding your health and adapt your approach accordingly. Keep in mind that effectively managing Hashimoto's isn't a straightforward journey. It demands flexibility and a readiness to adjust as your requirements evolve.

Customizing the Hashimoto's Protocol to suit your unique requirements is a continuous and ever-evolving journey. As you gain more knowledge about your body and its responses to various interventions, your needs may evolve over time. Remaining receptive and adaptable to new information or changes in your condition is important.

This adaptability is a strong point, not a flaw. By adopting a flexible approach and being open to making necessary changes, you have the ability to develop a customized method for effectively managing Hashimoto's that enhances your overall health, well-being, and quality of life. Have confidence in your capacity to navigate this journey, and always keep in mind that you possess knowledge about your own body. With the proper resources, assistance, and a positive outlook, it is possible to successfully control Hashimoto's and lead a lively and well-balanced life.

Conclusion

In this chapter, we've explored the Hashimoto's Protocol, a strategic approach to managing Hashimoto's Thyroiditis that is rooted in understanding the condition at its core. We delved into the foundational principles of the protocol, highlighting the importance of addressing root causes, restoring gut health, balancing hormones, reducing inflammation, supporting detoxification, and optimizing nutrition and lifestyle. Each of these elements plays a crucial role in creating a comprehensive plan that not only manages symptoms but also promotes overall wellness.

Equally important is the emphasis on personalization. We discussed how tailoring the Hashimoto's Protocol to individual needs is essential for its success. Recognizing that each person's experience with Hashimoto is unique, the protocol encourages a flexible and dynamic approach, one that adapts to the changing needs and circumstances of the individual. By focusing on personalized strategies, individuals can address their specific triggers, support their unique biochemistry, and create a path to healing that resonates with their body's needs.

As we move forward, the insights gained from this chapter provide a solid foundation for exploring the specific steps and actions that can be taken to implement the Hashimoto's Protocol effectively. Armed with this knowledge, you are now ready to take the next step in your journey, crafting a personalized plan that empowers you to live a healthier, more vibrant life despite the challenges of Hashimoto's. This journey is not just about managing a condition; it's about reclaiming your health and embracing a proactive approach to wellness.

4

Medical and Holistic Treatment Options

"Health is not just about the absence of disease; it's about achieving a balance of body, mind, and spirit."

Managing Hashimoto's Thyroiditis requires a multifaceted approach that goes beyond simply addressing symptoms. As an autoimmune condition, Hashimoto's affects the entire body, intertwining with various systems and influencing overall health. This complexity demands a treatment strategy that is both comprehensive and flexible, combining the strengths of conventional medicine with the insights and practices of holistic therapies. By doing so, we not only aim to manage the disease more effectively but also to enhance overall well-being and quality of life.

In this chapter, we explore the spectrum of medical and holistic treatment options available for managing Hashimoto's Thyroiditis. We begin with an in-depth look at conventional treatments, focusing on the role of medications and therapies that form the backbone of medical management. From thyroid hormone replacement to immune-modulating drugs, these treatments provide essential support for those navigating the challenges of this condition. However, to fully address the needs of individuals with Hashimoto's, it is equally important to consider integrative approaches that incorporate alternative medicine. By combining Western and alternative therapies, we can create a personalized treatment plan that addresses the root causes of the disease, reduces inflammation, and promotes overall health. This chapter will guide you through the various options, empowering you to make informed decisions about your health journey.

4.1. Conventional Treatments: Medications and Therapies

Understanding the conventional medical options available is crucial when navigating the treatment landscape for Hashimoto's Thyroiditis. These treatments focus on medications and therapies to effectively manage symptoms, restore thyroid hormone levels, and halt the progression of the disease. Conventional treatments serve as a vital base for countless individuals who are navigating Hashimoto's. These treatments don't provide a cure, but they do offer much-needed relief from the overwhelming symptoms and assist in maintaining a sense of normalcy in day-to-day life.

The Importance of Thyroid Hormone Replacement

Thyroid hormone replacement therapy forms the foundation of conventional treatment for Hashimoto's. This approach focuses on the key characteristic of the disease: the decreased production of thyroid hormones caused by the immune system's attack on the thyroid gland. When the thyroid's ability to produce essential hormones decreases, it becomes necessary to supplement in order to restore balance and support the body's metabolic functions.

Levothyroxine is the most frequently prescribed medication for thyroid hormone replacement. It is a synthetic version of thyroxine (T4), which is the main hormone produced by the thyroid gland. Levothyroxine is formulated to imitate the natural T4 hormone, ensuring a consistent and reliable dosage that can be converted into the more potent triiodothyronine (T3) by the body when necessary. It is recommended to take this medication once daily, preferably in the morning on an empty stomach, for best absorption and effectiveness.

Initial doses of levothyroxine are meticulously determined, taking into account various factors including age, weight, the extent of hormone deficiency, and any additional underlying health conditions. Regular blood tests are essential for monitoring TSH (thyroid-stimulating hormone) and T4 levels once a patient starts therapy. These tests help ensure that the medication is effectively restoring hormone balance without leading to hyperthyroidism, or an overactive thyroid. Dosage adjustments may be required over time, particularly in light of changes in weight, health status, or life circumstances like pregnancy.

The Significance of Personalized Dosage

It's important to acknowledge that thyroid hormone replacement therapy is not a universal solution, even for patients with Hashimoto's. Although levothyroxine is commonly prescribed, it may not be suitable for everyone. Every individual's body has its own unique response to medication, and determining the appropriate dosage requires both time and patience. Certain people may continue to have symptoms even when their TSH and T4 levels are normal, indicating that their body's conversion of T4 to T3 may not be optimal.

Considering a combination therapy that includes both levothyroxine (T4) and liothyronine (T3) may be an option in such cases. Liothyronine is a synthetic form of T3, which is considered to be the more active thyroid hormone. By combining these medications, certain patients who experience discomfort on T4-only therapy can find relief. This approach offers a more balanced solution that closely resembles the natural hormone production of a healthy thyroid. Nevertheless, this treatment necessitates meticulous supervision and should be overseen by a well-informed healthcare professional to prevent possible adverse reactions, like rapid heartbeats or feelings of unease, linked to elevated T3 levels.

Monitoring and managing side effects

Just like any medication, thyroid hormone replacement therapy has its own set of potential side effects and things to consider. Patients should be well-informed about these matters and maintain open communication with their healthcare provider to ensure their condition is managed optimally. Typical side effects of thyroid hormone replacement may manifest as hyperthyroidism symptoms, including a heightened heart rate, feelings of anxiety, difficulty sleeping, and weight loss. These symptoms commonly suggest that the dosage may require adjustment.

On the other hand, if the dosage is insufficient, symptoms of hypothyroidism, such as fatigue, weight gain, and depression, may continue to be present. Consistent follow-up appointments and blood tests are essential for optimizing the medication and ensuring it effectively relieves symptoms without any potential health complications. It's important for patients to be mindful of possible interactions between thyroid hormone replacement therapy and other medications. For instance, taking calcium or iron supplements too closely together can hinder absorption.

Addressing Inflammation and Immune Response

Although thyroid hormone replacement therapy is effective in managing the symptoms of hypothyroidism in Hashimoto, it does not target the root cause of the autoimmune response that triggers the disease. For this reason, certain patients may also receive prescriptions for medications that help control inflammation or regulate the immune system. These treatments are usually considered when there is noticeable inflammation or when other autoimmune conditions coexist with Hashimoto's.

Nonsteroidal anti-inflammatory drugs (NSAIDs) such as ibuprofen or naproxen can be effective in reducing inflammation and providing pain relief for cases of severe thyroid inflammation. In more severe instances, doctors may recommend corticosteroids to help control the immune system and alleviate inflammation. Nevertheless, these medications are typically prescribed for a limited duration because of their potential side effects and the possibility of developing long-term complications, such as decreased bone density and heightened vulnerability to infections.

Impact of Selenium and Other Supplements

Aside from medications, specific supplements might be considered as part of conventional treatment plans for Hashimoto's. Research has demonstrated that selenium, a vital trace mineral for thyroid health, can effectively lower thyroid antibody levels and enhance overall thyroid function in certain individuals. It is believed that this effect is a result of selenium's involvement in the conversion of T4 to T3 and its capacity to decrease oxidative stress in the thyroid gland.

It is advisable to consult with a healthcare provider before beginning any supplement regimen, as they can provide guidance on the appropriate dosage of selenium for individuals with Hashimoto's. A common recommendation is a daily dosage of 200 micrograms. Supplements like zinc, vitamin D, and omega-3 fatty acids can also contribute to thyroid function and boost overall immune health. However, it's important to personalize their inclusion in a treatment plan according to individual needs and deficiencies.

The Importance of Patient Education and Advocacy

Understanding and advocating for your own health is crucial when it comes to managing Hashimoto's with conventional treatments. Having a thorough understanding of medications, including their purposes and potential side effects, allows patients to play an active role in managing their health. It's critical for individuals with Hashimoto's to feel at ease when discussing their symptoms and concerns with their healthcare provider, and to confidently advocate for any necessary adjustments to their treatment plan.

It is important to advise patients to maintain a comprehensive log of their symptoms, medication dosages, and any potential side effects they may encounter. This information is extremely valuable during follow-up appointments, enabling healthcare providers to make well-informed decisions about treatment adjustments and ensuring optimal effectiveness of the chosen therapy.

The drawbacks of traditional treatment methods

Although conventional treatments are helpful for managing Hashimoto's Thyroiditis, it is important to recognize their limitations. Although thyroid hormone replacement therapy is successful in restoring hormone levels, it does not provide a cure for the underlying autoimmune disease or prevent the immune system from targeting the thyroid. Unfortunately, even with the right medication, some patients may still experience symptoms or see their condition worsen.

This acknowledgment underscores the significance of adopting a holistic and diverse method in the management of Hashimoto's. It involves combining traditional treatments with other approaches that target the underlying causes of the disease, promote overall well-being, and improve quality of life.

Conventional treatments provide a solid basis for managing Hashimoto's Thyroiditis, offering hormone replacement and relief from symptoms. For optimal results, it is important to consider these treatments as part of a comprehensive and holistic approach to health. Through the integration of conventional therapies, personalized lifestyle modifications, nutritional support, and stress management, individuals with Hashimoto's can develop a comprehensive plan to enhance their overall health and well-being.

Throughout this book, we will delve into the integration of conventional treatments with holistic and alternative approaches.

By doing so, we aim to provide you with a comprehensive strategy that will empower you to effectively manage Hashimoto's and live a vibrant, healthy life.

4.2. Integrative Approaches: Combining Western and Alternative Medicine

Managing Hashimoto's Thyroiditis requires finding a delicate balance between conventional and alternative medicine, which can have a transformative impact. An integrative approach recognizes the importance of conventional treatments such as medication, but also acknowledges that they may not fully address all aspects of the disease or meet the unique needs of each individual. Through the integration of Western medical practices and alternative therapies, patients can experience the advantages of a well-rounded approach that focuses on both symptom relief and overall well-being. This comprehensive strategy aims to address the underlying causes of health issues and improve quality of life.

The Philosophy Behind Integrative Medicine

Integrative medicine recognizes that healing encompasses various aspects of well-being, including physical, emotional, mental, and spiritual aspects. It highlights the importance of the patient's active participation in their health journey and aims to incorporate the most effective evidence-based practices from both Western and alternative medicine. This approach does not involve favoring one method over another. Instead, it focuses on developing a harmonious plan that utilizes the unique advantages of various modalities to deliver a comprehensive and tailored treatment.

Integrative medicine acknowledges the complexity of autoimmune diseases like Hashimoto's and emphasizes the need for a nuanced approach. Although thyroid hormone replacement is successful in managing the thyroid hormone deficiency associated with Hashimoto's, it does not target the root autoimmune process or the lifestyle factors that can worsen the condition. Integrative medicine addresses the need for therapies that can help reduce inflammation, regulate the immune system, enhance gut health, and promote the body's innate healing abilities.

Acupuncture and Traditional Chinese Medicine

Acupuncture is widely recognized as a highly effective alternative therapy in the field of integrative medicine, closely associated with Traditional Chinese Medicine (TCM). Acupuncture utilizes the insertion of fine needles into precise points on the body to enhance energy flow, alleviate discomfort, and facilitate the body's natural healing processes. Acupuncture can provide significant relief for individuals with Hashimoto's, helping to manage symptoms such as fatigue, pain, and stress.

Acupuncture is thought to promote the balance of the body's energy and improve the circulation of blood and nutrients to important organs like the thyroid. It can also help regulate the immune response, potentially reducing inflammation and autoimmune activity. There is evidence to support the idea that regular acupuncture treatments may have a positive impact on thyroid function and overall well-being in individuals with Hashimoto's. In addition, acupuncture has been found to promote relaxation and reduce stress, which is important for individuals dealing with autoimmune conditions. This is because stress can have a significant impact on immune function.

TCM provides herbal therapies that can help support thyroid health and balance the immune system. Herbs like astragalus, rehmannia, and licorice root, have long been revered in Traditional Chinese Medicine (TCM) for their potent properties. These botanicals play a crucial role in ancient herbal remedies, contributing to a holistic approach to health that aims to restore balance and harmony to the body's energies. For individuals dealing with Hashimoto's Thyroiditis, these herbs provide potential advantages that go beyond traditional treatments, targeting the underlying causes of the condition and supporting overall health.

Astragalus is commonly known as a "adaptogen," a natural substance believed to assist the body in coping with stress and promoting balance in bodily functions. In traditional Chinese medicine, astragalus is renowned for its capacity to strengthen the immune system, boost energy levels, and shield against the detrimental impacts of stress. This herb is highly regarded for its remarkable capacity to regulate the immune system, whether by boosting its activity or soothing it when necessary. For individuals with Hashimoto's, astragalus can provide gentle regulation of immune function. It helps support the body's defenses without causing excessive stimulation of the immune response, which may help reduce the autoimmune activity associated with Hashimoto's.

In addition to its immune-modulating properties, astragalus is highly regarded for its anti-inflammatory and antioxidant effects. With its ability to reduce inflammation and protect cells from oxidative damage, astragalus can effectively address the underlying processes that contribute to the progression of the disease.

Rehmannia, known as the "kidney tonic," has a rich history in TCM for its ability to nourish and harmonize the body's internal energies. This herb is commonly used to support the health of the kidneys and adrenal glands, which play a vital role in hormone production and stress response. According to traditional Chinese medicine, the kidneys are believed to be the foundation of vitality and essential for maintaining good health and longevity.

Rehmannia's benefits are especially relevant for individuals with Hashimoto's. Hashimoto's is frequently accompanied by adrenal fatigue as a result of prolonged stress and the body's ongoing effort to maintain equilibrium in the face of autoimmune activity. Rehmannia is beneficial for nourishing the adrenal glands, which in turn supports the production of cortisol and other essential hormones that play a vital role in stress management. Rehmannia has the potential to enhance energy levels, boost resilience, and promote optimal functioning of the endocrine system.

Rehmannia is known for its anti-inflammatory and immune-modulating properties, which can be beneficial in managing Hashimoto's. It has a cooling and calming effect on the immune system, which helps to reduce inflammation and prevent damage to the thyroid. In addition, rehmannia has been discovered to possess neuroprotective properties, making it potentially advantageous for those who are dealing with cognitive symptoms, like brain fog, commonly associated with thyroid dysfunction.

Another herb highly valued in TCM is **licorice root**, known for its sweet flavor and potent medicinal properties. Licorice root is recognized for its harmonizing properties in herbal formulas, which contribute to balancing the effects of other herbs and amplifying their efficacy. However, its advantages extend well beyond this supportive function.

Licorice root is known for its ability to promote adrenal health, just like rehmannia. Licorice contains compounds that can extend the activity of cortisol, the body's main stress hormone, by inhibiting its breakdown. This can be especially helpful for individuals with Hashimoto's who are dealing with adrenal fatigue, as it aids in maintaining consistent cortisol levels and preventing the energy crashes commonly associated with low adrenal function.

Licorice root is well-known for its impressive anti-inflammatory properties. This compound has been proven to have anti-inflammatory properties and can help regulate the immune system. For individuals with Hashimoto's, licorice has the potential to calm the overactive immune response that targets the thyroid gland. This may lead to a slower progression of the disease and a reduction in symptoms.

In addition, licorice root has a calming impact on the digestive system. This herb is highly beneficial for individuals with Hashimoto's who are also experiencing gastrointestinal issues such as leaky gut syndrome, as it aids in the healing and protection of the stomach and intestinal lining. Supporting gut health is important for maintaining a well-functioning immune system. Licorice root can help with this by indirectly promoting immune balance.

Exploring Nutritional Therapy and Functional Medicine

Integrative medicine places great emphasis on the importance of nutritional therapy, especially when it comes to effectively managing autoimmune diseases such as Hashimoto's. Research continues to highlight the significant impact of diet on the immune system, inflammation reduction, and thyroid function support.

Using a functional medicine approach, comprehensive testing can be conducted to identify potential nutrient deficiencies, food sensitivities, and other imbalances that may play a role in Hashimoto's. Using the research findings, a customized nutrition plan is created, emphasizing the inclusion of anti-inflammatory foods, nutrient-rich choices, and the avoidance of potential triggers such as gluten, dairy, and processed foods. This approach focuses on the inclusion of specific nutrients to support thyroid health and immune function. Foods rich in selenium, zinc, iodine, and omega-3 fatty acids are emphasized for their beneficial effects.

In addition to diet, functional medicine may also incorporate targeted supplementation to address specific deficiencies or support the body's natural detoxification processes. Supplements such as probiotics, vitamin D, and antioxidants have been shown to promote a healthy gut microbiome, reduce oxidative stress, and boost immune health.

Mind-Body Medicine: Stress Management and Emotional Well-being

An integrative approach to Hashimoto's also emphasizes the importance of mind-body medicine, acknowledging the significant influence that stress and emotional well-being can have on physical health. Chronic stress can worsen autoimmune diseases by triggering inflammation and disrupting the delicate balance of hormones. Thus, mastering stress management techniques becomes essential in effectively managing Hashimoto's.

Engaging in activities like mindfulness meditation, yoga, and tai chi has been proven to effectively alleviate stress, boost mood, and promote a sense of well-being. These techniques can help you relax, decrease anxiety, and regulate your body's stress response. Practicing mindfulness meditation entails directing your attention to the present moment and nurturing a non-judgmental understanding of your thoughts and emotions. This technique can assist individuals with Hashimoto's in developing a greater awareness of their bodies and improving their ability to handle stress and emotional triggers.

Practicing yoga and tai chi, with their focus on physical movement, breath awareness, and mindfulness, can offer great benefits to those with Hashimoto's. These practices can enhance flexibility, balance, and strength, while also promoting a feeling of tranquility and serenity. In addition, the social aspects of group classes can offer a strong sense of community and support, which can be incredibly valuable for individuals facing the difficulties of a chronic illness.

Integrating Conventional and Alternative Therapies

An integrative approach excels in its capacity to blend conventional and alternative therapies, resulting in a comprehensive plan that caters to all aspects of health. This approach acknowledges the importance of medications such as thyroid hormone replacement in the management of Hashimoto's, understanding that they are only a part of the overall solution. Through the integration of alternative therapies that target the underlying causes of the disease, alleviate inflammation, and promote overall wellness, individuals can attain a more harmonized and efficient approach to managing their condition.

In order to effectively incorporate these therapies, it is important to collaborate with a healthcare team that is receptive to both conventional and alternative methods and can assist you in developing a unified strategy. It's crucial to maintain open lines of communication with all your healthcare providers so they can collaborate effectively and provide you with the best possible care. This comprehensive approach guarantees that every aspect of your health is taken into account and that your treatment plan is customized to meet your individual requirements.

Ultimately, the aim of an integrative approach is to not only manage Hashimoto's, but to thrive despite it. By adopting a comprehensive approach that considers all facets of your health—physical, emotional, and mental—you can improve your overall well-being and experience a higher standard of living.

Conclusion

In this chapter, we have delved into the diverse array of treatment options available for managing Hashimoto's Thyroiditis, underscoring the importance of a comprehensive, integrative approach. We began by exploring conventional treatments, including thyroid hormone replacement therapy and medications aimed at managing inflammation and modulating the immune system. These therapies help stabilize thyroid function and alleviate the symptoms associated with Hashimoto's.

However, we also recognized that conventional medicine, while essential, may not address all aspects of this complex autoimmune condition. This is where integrative approaches come into play, combining the best of Western and alternative medicine to create a holistic treatment plan. By incorporating therapies such as acupuncture, nutritional therapy, mind–body medicine, and herbal remedies, we can target the underlying causes of Hashimoto's, support overall health, and enhance the effectiveness of conventional treatments.

The ultimate goal of this chapter is to empower you with the knowledge and tools to create a personalized, integrative plan for managing Hashimoto's. By embracing both medical and holistic treatment options, you can navigate the complexities of this condition with confidence and take proactive steps toward achieving optimal health and well-being. As we continue this journey, we will further explore how to implement these strategies effectively, building on the foundation laid in this chapter to enhance your quality of life and overall health.

5

Nutritional Management for Hashimoto's

"Let food be thy medicine, and medicine be thy food." — Hippocrates

When it comes to managing Hashimoto's Thyroiditis, the food you choose to eat can be one of your most powerful allies. While medications and therapies play a vital role in managing symptoms, the right nutrition can provide the foundation for long-term health and well-being. In Hashimoto's, a well-balanced, nutrient-rich diet can help modulate the immune response, reduce inflammation, and support thyroid function.

This chapter delves into the critical role that nutrition plays in managing Hashimoto's. We will explore the essential nutrients that are vital for thyroid health and how they can impact your overall well-being. We'll also discuss which foods to avoid, as certain ingredients can exacerbate symptoms and trigger autoimmune reactions. Finally, we will provide sample meal plans and recipes that are not only nutritious but also delicious, demonstrating that eating for thyroid health can be both satisfying and enjoyable. With the right nutritional approach, you can take significant steps towards managing Hashimoto's and enhancing your quality of life.

5.1. Essential Nutrients and Their Impact on Thyroid Health

The connection between nutrition and thyroid health is incredibly significant and complex. Understanding the role of essential nutrients is crucial for those managing Hashimoto's Thyroiditis.

In order to operate at its best, the body depends on a consistent intake of essential nutrients that promote the production of hormones, boost the immune system, and maintain cellular well-being. When there is a lack or imbalance of these nutrients, it can negatively impact the thyroid's functioning, making the symptoms of Hashimoto's worse and potentially speeding up the progression of the disease.

The Power of Iodine: A Double-Edged Sword

Iodine is widely recognized as a vital nutrient for maintaining optimal thyroid function. Iodine supports the synthesis of thyroid hormones, specifically thyroxine (T4) and triiodothyronine (T3). Insufficient iodine can hinder the thyroid's ability to produce sufficient levels of T4 and T3, resulting in hypothyroidism. In regions where iodine deficiency is prevalent, goiter may develop as the thyroid gland enlarges in an effort to compensate for the insufficient hormone production.

For individuals with Hashimoto's, it is important to be cautious when it comes to iodine intake. Excessive iodine intake can worsen autoimmune activity, despite the fact that the thyroid needs iodine. Excessive iodine has the potential to trigger or exacerbate the autoimmune attack on the thyroid gland, which can result in heightened inflammation and damage to the thyroid. It is crucial to maintain a well-balanced intake that adequately supports thyroid function without worsening the autoimmune process. It is key to collaborate with a healthcare provider to determine the ideal iodine levels for your individual requirements, as this balance is intricate and differs from person to person.

Selenium: A Powerful Protector for the Thyroid

Selenium is an essential nutrient for maintaining thyroid health, known for its protective properties that help shield the thyroid. This essential mineral plays a crucial role in the conversion of T4 to the more potent T3 hormone, which is responsible for the majority of thyroid hormone activity in the body. Moreover, it is important to note that selenium has a vital role in the production of glutathione peroxidase. This antioxidant enzyme is responsible for safeguarding the thyroid gland from oxidative stress and inflammation, which are particularly heightened in individuals with Hashimoto's.

Several studies have demonstrated the potential of selenium supplementation in reducing thyroid antibody levels in individuals with Hashimoto's, indicating its ability to regulate the autoimmune response. In addition, the antioxidant properties of selenium can help reduce the harm caused by chronic inflammation, providing further protection for the thyroid gland. Ensuring sufficient selenium intake is vital for managing Hashimoto's and promoting thyroid health. Some examples of foods that are high in selenium are Brazil nuts, sunflower seeds, and fatty fish such as sardines.

Zinc

Zinc is an essential nutrient that plays a crucial role in supporting thyroid function and maintaining a healthy immune system. Similar to selenium, zinc also contributes to the conversion of T4 to T3, which aids in the regulation of thyroid hormone levels within the body. Zinc supports the synthesis of thyroid-stimulating hormone (TSH), which is produced by the pituitary gland to regulate thyroid function.

In addition to its involvement in hormone production, zinc plays a vital role in supporting a healthy immune system. It aids in the function of immune cells and plays a role in regulating the immune response, which is especially beneficial for those with autoimmune conditions such as Hashimoto's. Research has shown that a lack of zinc can negatively impact the immune system, potentially worsening the autoimmune assault on the thyroid. Ensuring sufficient zinc intake through diet or supplementation can contribute to maintaining immune balance and safeguarding thyroid health. Excellent dietary sources of zinc are shellfish, beef, eggs, and oysters.

Vitamin D: Regulating the Immune System

Research has demonstrated the importance of Vitamin D in immune regulation and its impact on autoimmune diseases like Hashimoto's. Understanding the role of Vitamin D in the immune system is crucial in preventing an excessive immune response that may result in harm to the body's tissues. Studies have linked insufficient vitamin D levels to a higher likelihood of developing autoimmune thyroid diseases. Additionally, research suggests that taking vitamin D supplements can help lower thyroid antibody levels in certain individuals with Hashimoto's.

In addition to its role in modulating the immune system, vitamin D plays a crucial role in maintaining calcium metabolism and promoting healthy bones. This is particularly significant for individuals with thyroid disorders, as their bone health can be impacted. It is important to note that adequate sun exposure is necessary for the synthesis of Vitamin D in the skin. However, certain factors such as limited sun exposure during winter months or residing in higher latitudes can lead to insufficient levels of this essential vitamin. Given the circumstances, it may be necessary for many individuals with Hashimoto's to consider vitamin D supplementation in order to maintain adequate levels and support thyroid health.

Magnesium

Many people tend to overlook the importance of magnesium when it comes to thyroid health. However, this mineral is actually quite important in maintaining hormonal balance and promoting overall well-being. It is well known that magnesium plays a crucial role in regulating the hypothalamic-pituitary-thyroid (HPT) axis. This axis is responsible for overseeing the production and release of thyroid hormones. Having sufficient magnesium levels is essential for the conversion of T4 to T3, as well as for the production of ATP, the cell's energy source that is vital for all metabolic functions.

Magnesium has a soothing impact on the nervous system, which can aid in alleviating stress and anxiety. These factors can worsen the symptoms of Hashimoto's. Chronic stress can lead to a decrease in magnesium levels, which can then contribute to a cycle of escalating stress and a decline in thyroid function. Making sure to get enough magnesium through your diet or by taking supplements can help break this cycle, promoting a healthy thyroid and increasing your ability to handle stress. Include leafy greens, nuts, and whole grains in your diet for a good source of magnesium.

Iron: Maximizing Oxygen Delivery and Metabolic Efficiency

Iron is a nutrient that plays a vital role in maintaining thyroid health. It is an important component of hemoglobin, the protein found in red blood cells that transports oxygen to tissues in the body. Proper oxygen delivery is essential for all metabolic processes, including those occurring in the thyroid gland. Iron plays a vital role in the synthesis of thyroid peroxidase (TPO), an enzyme that is essential for the production of thyroid hormones.

Iron deficiency is a common issue, particularly among women, and can worsen symptoms of hypothyroidism, like fatigue and cognitive impairment. It is critical to maintain optimal thyroid function and overall energy levels by ensuring adequate iron intake through diet or supplementation. Nevertheless, it is important to keep a close eye on iron levels and collaborate with a healthcare provider, as excessive iron supplementation can have detrimental effects. Excellent dietary sources of iron consist of red meat, poultry, and fish.

Omega-3 Fatty Acids: Decreasing Inflammation

Omega-3 fatty acids, which can be found in fatty fish such as salmon and mackerel are well-known for their anti-inflammatory properties. Chronic inflammation has a big role in Hashimoto's, leading to damage in the thyroid tissue and the advancement of the disease. Omega-3 fatty acids help reduce inflammation by regulating the production of inflammatory cytokines and maintaining the health of cell membranes.

Including omega-3-rich foods in your diet or using a high-quality fish oil supplement can be beneficial in reducing the inflammatory response in Hashimoto's, safeguarding the thyroid gland, and promoting overall well-being. These fatty acids are beneficial for brain health and cardiovascular function, making them a valuable addition to any diet aimed at managing autoimmune conditions.

Having a thorough understanding of the role that essential nutrients play in maintaining thyroid health is vital when it comes to effectively managing Hashimoto's Thyroiditis. It is essential to maintain a proper diet and consider individual needs and potential interactions to support thyroid function and overall well-being. With a comprehensive perspective on nutrition, individuals with Hashimoto's can establish a solid basis for optimal health. This approach highlights the importance of consuming high-quality, diverse, and balanced foods, leading to a reduction in symptoms and an improvement in overall quality of life.

When delving into the realm of nutrition and its impact on managing Hashimoto's, it's important to keep in mind that individual needs vary greatly. Collaborating with a healthcare provider to track nutrient levels and customize your diet can lead to optimal results. With the right balance of vital nutrients and thoughtful lifestyle decisions, effectively managing this intricate autoimmune condition and preserving overall well-being becomes possible.

5.2. Avoiding Foods That Worsen Symptoms

Proper management of Hashimoto's Thyroiditis involves harnessing the potential of your diet as a valuable tool. Proper nutrition is essential for maintaining thyroid health and promoting a balanced immune system while also helping to minimize inflammation. When dealing with Hashimoto's, it's crucial to not only include the necessary nutrients but also steer clear of foods that can worsen symptoms, provoke autoimmune reactions, or disrupt thyroid function. The objective is to establish a conducive internal environment that facilitates healing, reduces strain on the thyroid, and avoids unwarranted immune system activation.

The Impact of Gluten on Autoimmune Thyroid Disease

Gluten is a frequently discussed dietary trigger in Hashimoto's management. For individuals with autoimmune diseases, gluten, a protein found in wheat, barley, and rye, can pose some challenges. Consuming gluten can lead to increased intestinal permeability, commonly known as "leaky gut," especially for individuals with Hashimoto's. During this condition, the lining of the intestines becomes more permeable, which results in the entry of undigested food particles and toxins into the bloodstream. This can potentially trigger an immune response, which can further worsen inflammation and contribute to the autoimmune attack on the thyroid gland.

In addition, the molecular structure of gluten bears resemblance to that of the thyroid gland. This phenomenon, referred to as molecular mimicry, can lead to the immune system confusing thyroid tissue with gluten and erroneously launching an attack on it, exacerbating the symptoms of Hashimoto's. Numerous people with Hashimoto's have experienced a decrease in symptoms like fatigue, mental fogginess, and joint discomfort by removing gluten from their diets. While not everyone with Hashimoto's experiences gluten sensitivity, it is commonly advised to experiment with a gluten-free diet to determine if it alleviates symptoms.

The Impact of Dairy on Inflammation and Autoimmunity

Dairy can be a common trigger for individuals with Hashimoto's. Although dairy products are packed with essential nutrients such as calcium and vitamin D, they may cause inflammation in certain people. Some individuals may experience difficulty digesting dairy proteins, such as casein and whey, which could potentially lead to an immune response, particularly in those who have sensitivities or intolerances. This immune response can result in heightened inflammation throughout the body, which may affect the thyroid gland.

Furthermore, dairy has the potential to trigger inflammation and exacerbate digestive problems like bloating, gas, and diarrhea, which are frequently experienced by individuals with Hashimoto's. These digestive issues can worsen gut health, triggering a cycle of inflammation and immune system activation that can make thyroid symptoms worse. Individuals with Hashimoto's may experience symptom reduction and improved well-being by eliminating dairy from their diet, just like they would with gluten. It is crucial to understand how your body responds to dairy products and make necessary adjustments to your diet, as dairy sensitivity can differ greatly among individuals.

The Link Between Soy and Thyroid Function

Soy is frequently mentioned when discussing thyroid health. Soy contains goitrogens, which can disrupt thyroid hormone production by affecting the thyroid's ability to utilize iodine. For individuals with Hashimoto's, this can pose a significant challenge since their thyroid function is already compromised. In addition, soy is frequently genetically modified and heavily processed, which can exacerbate its potential to disrupt thyroid function and promote inflammation.

For certain individuals with Hashimoto's, the consumption of soy may result in elevated levels of thyroid-stimulating hormone (TSH), suggesting that the thyroid is exerting more effort to produce sufficient hormones. These symptoms of hypothyroidism can become worse, leading to fatigue, weight gain, and depression. Although some individuals may be able to tolerate moderate consumption of soy, it is generally advised to limit or avoid soy products, especially highly processed forms such as soy protein isolates. This is to promote thyroid health and reduce the chances of exacerbating symptoms.

The Hidden Dangers of Sugar and Processed Foods

The prevalence of sugar and processed foods in the modern diet is concerning, particularly for individuals with Hashimoto's. Consuming excessive amounts of sugar and refined carbohydrates can contribute to blood sugar imbalances, weight gain, and insulin resistance. These factors can worsen thyroid dysfunction and autoimmune activity. When blood sugar levels fluctuate frequently, it can strain the adrenal glands and potentially disrupt hormonal balance, which can have negative effects on thyroid health.

Processed foods are frequently packed with additives, preservatives, and artificial ingredients that have the potential to cause inflammation and immune reactions. These foods are usually lacking in important nutrients and packed with unhealthy fats, sugars, and salt, which can lead to a diet that promotes inflammation and is not beneficial for thyroid and overall health. To promote better health and support your thyroid function, it's important for those with Hashimoto's to steer clear of processed foods and added sugars. This can help reduce inflammation and stabilize blood sugar levels.

The Effects of Nightshade Vegetables on Autoimmune Diseases

Some people with autoimmune diseases like Hashimoto's may find nightshade vegetables, such as tomatoes, potatoes, eggplants, and peppers, to be potentially problematic for their health. These vegetables contain alkaloids, which are naturally occurring compounds that may cause inflammation and immune responses in certain individuals. Some individuals may experience relief from joint pain, inflammation, and other autoimmune symptoms by excluding nightshade vegetables from their diet, although this is not the case for everyone with

Hashimoto's.

If you think nightshades could be playing a role in your symptoms, you might want to try removing them from your diet for a while and then gradually reintroducing them to observe how your body reacts. This approach can be valuable in identifying potential food sensitivities and guiding dietary choices to support thyroid health.

The Effects of Goitrogenic Foods on Thyroid Health

Certain foods, including cruciferous vegetables like broccoli, cauliflower, and Brussels sprouts, have the potential to disrupt thyroid hormone production by affecting iodine uptake. Although these vegetables are packed with nutrients and offer numerous health advantages, their goitrogenic properties may be worrisome for individuals with Hashimoto's, particularly if consumed in excessive quantities or in their raw state. When vegetables are cooked, their goitrogenic effects are reduced, which can make them a safer option for individuals with thyroid issues.

It's worth mentioning that not everyone with Hashimoto's has to completely avoid goitrogenic foods. Actually, a lot of individuals can consume them without any adverse effects on thyroid function, particularly when they are prepared and consumed in reasonable amounts. It's important to pay attention to how your body reacts and collaborate with a healthcare provider to find the most suitable approach for your specific requirements.

Alcohol's Impact on Autoimmunity and Thyroid Health

Alcohol can greatly affect the health of the thyroid and the functioning of the immune system, especially for those with Hashimoto's disease. Drinking alcohol can worsen inflammation, disrupt the health of your gut, and harm your liver function, all of which can make your Hashimoto's symptoms worse. Alcohol can disrupt the metabolism of thyroid hormones and exacerbate hormonal imbalances, which can further compromise thyroid function.

It is generally recommended for individuals with Hashimoto's to limit or avoid alcohol consumption in order to minimize its effects on the thyroid and immune system. If you decide to consume alcohol, it's important to practice moderation and pay attention to your body's reactions. Being mindful of symptoms and making appropriate adjustments to alcohol consumption can contribute to maintaining thyroid health and overall well-being.

Developing a Customized Diet Plan for Hashimoto's

Managing Hashimoto's requires a careful approach to food choices. It is critical to avoid foods that exacerbate symptoms, while also developing a personalized diet that caters to your specific needs. Every individual has unique nutritional needs, and what may be effective for one person might not yield the same results for someone else. By paying close attention to how your body reacts to various foods and making necessary changes, you can develop a diet that is beneficial for your thyroid health, minimizes inflammation, and enhances your overall well-being.

Collaborating with a healthcare provider or nutritionist who has expertise in Hashimoto's can offer valuable assistance in pinpointing possible dietary triggers and developing a personalized plan that suits your specific requirements. With keen observation, thorough testing, and a willingness to adapt, one can discover a dietary approach that effectively manages symptoms and promotes overall well-being.

Managing Hashimoto's through diet is not about restriction; it's about making educated decisions that align with your body's needs and your health objectives. By making conscious choices about the foods you consume and prioritizing nutrient-rich, anti-inflammatory options, you can establish a strong basis for promoting healing and overall wellness. Every individual's path to wellness is distinct, but armed with accurate knowledge and a strong support system, you can confidently navigate this journey and attain a higher standard of living.

As you delve into the realm of nutrition and its impact on managing Hashimoto's, it's important to keep in mind that your body can provide valuable insights. Pay attention to the signals your body sends, respect its needs, and be willing to make changes as you gain more knowledge about what suits you best. By dedicating yourself to your well-being and being persistent, you can discover a dietary strategy that promotes thyroid health and allows you to flourish.

5.3. Sample Meal Plans and Recipes

Creating a nourishing diet that supports thyroid health and manages Hashimoto's symptoms involves more than just understanding which foods to include and which to avoid. It's about bringing this knowledge into the kitchen, crafting meals that are not only healthful but also satisfying and delicious. A thoughtfully designed meal plan can help guide your daily choices, ensuring that you're consistently providing your body with the nutrients it needs while steering clear of potential triggers. In this section, we'll explore a variety of sample meal plans and recipes that embody the principles of nutritional management for Hashimoto's, emphasizing balance, variety, and flavor.

A Day of Balanced Nutrition

A well-rounded diet for managing Hashimoto's incorporates plenty of whole foods, rich in essential nutrients, while avoiding inflammatory ingredients that could exacerbate symptoms. The following sample meal plan offers a snapshot of a day designed to optimize thyroid health and overall well-being.

Breakfast: Omega-Packed Green Smoothie

Starting your day with a nutrient-dense smoothie can be a great way to fuel your body and support thyroid health. A green smoothie loaded with omega-3 fatty acids, vitamins, and minerals helps reduce inflammation and provide energy.

- Ingredients: 1 cup unsweetened almond milk, 1 handful of spinach, ½ avocado, 1 tablespoon chia seeds, 1 tablespoon ground flaxseeds, 1 teaspoon spirulina powder, ½ cup frozen blueberries, and 1 scoop of collagen protein powder.

- Instructions: Blend all ingredients in a high-speed blender until smooth and creamy. The avocado provides a creamy texture, while the chia and flaxseeds offer a boost of fiber and omega-3s. Spirulina adds an extra punch of protein and micronutrients, and the blueberries deliver antioxidants.

Mid-Morning Snack: Sliced Apples with Almond Butter

For a simple and satisfying snack, try pairing a sliced apple with a tablespoon of almond butter. This combination provides a good balance of carbohydrates, healthy fats, and protein, helping to keep your blood sugar stable and your energy levels steady.

Lunch: Grilled Salmon Salad with Lemon-Tahini Dressing

A hearty salad featuring grilled salmon offers a wealth of bene-fits for those managing Hashimoto's. Salmon is an excellent source of omega-3 fatty acids, which help reduce inflammation and support immune health. Pairing it with a variety of colorful vegetables adds fiber, vitamins, and minerals to the meal.

- Ingredients: 4-6 oz grilled salmon, mixed greens (such as kale, spinach, and arugula), ½ cup cherry tomatoes, ¼ cup sliced cucumbers, ¼ cup shredded carrots, ¼ avocado, and 2 tablespoons pumpkin seeds.

- Lemon-Tahini Dressing: Whisk together 2 tablespoons tahini, 1 tablespoon lemon juice, 1 tablespoon olive oil, 1 clove minced garlic, salt, and pepper to taste.

- Instructions: Arrange the greens on a plate and top with the vegetables, avocado, and pumpkin seeds. Place the grilled salmon on top and drizzle with lemon-tahini dressing. This meal provides a mix of healthy fats, protein, and antioxidants to support thyroid function and overall health.

Afternoon Snack: Turmeric and Ginger Golden Milk

Golden milk, made with turmeric and ginger, is a warming beverage that offers anti-inflammatory benefits. It's a comforting way to take a break in the afternoon while providing the body with powerful antioxidants.

- Ingredients: 1 cup unsweetened coconut milk, ½ teaspoon turmeric, ¼ teaspoon ground ginger, ¼ teaspoon cinnamon, 1 teaspoon honey or maple syrup (optional), and a pinch of black pepper.

- Instructions: In a small saucepan, whisk together the coconut milk, turmeric, ginger, cinnamon, and black pepper. Heat over medium heat until warm but not boiling. Add honey or maple syrup to taste, if desired. The combination of turmeric and ginger provides potent anti-inflammatory properties, while the coconut milk adds healthy fats.

Dinner: Baked Chicken Thighs with Roasted Vegetables

For dinner, baked chicken thighs paired with roasted vegetables create a comforting and nutrient-rich meal. Chicken thighs are a great source of protein, zinc, and selenium, all of which support thyroid health. Roasting the vegetables enhances their flavors and retains their nutritional value.

- Ingredients: 4 bone-in, skin-on chicken thighs, 1 tablespoon olive oil, salt, pepper, 1 teaspoon dried thyme, 2 cups chopped vegetables (such as sweet potatoes, carrots, zucchini, and bell peppers), 1 teaspoon smoked paprika.

- Instructions: Preheat the oven to 400°F. Rub the chicken thighs with olive oil, salt, pepper, and thyme. Place the chicken on a baking sheet and arrange the vegetables around the chicken. Sprinkle the vegetables with salt, pepper, and smoked paprika. Roast for 30-35 minutes or until the chicken is cooked through and the vegetables are tender. This meal is rich in protein and colorful vegetables, providing a balanced array of nutrients.

Dessert: Dark Chocolate Avocado Mousse

A creamy, decadent dessert can be both delicious and nutritious. This dark chocolate avocado mousse is packed with healthy fats and antioxidants, making it a guilt-free indulgence that supports thyroid health.

- Ingredients: 2 ripe avocados, ¼ cup unsweetened cocoa powder, ¼ cup maple syrup, 1 teaspoon vanilla extract, and a pinch of sea salt.

- Instructions: In a food processor, blend all ingredients until smooth and creamy. Chill for 30 minutes before serving. The avocados provide a rich texture and are full of healthy monounsaturated fats, while the cocoa powder adds antioxidants and depth of flavor.

Crafting Your Own Meal Plan

While the above meal plan offers a structured day of meals, the key to successful nutritional management of Hashimoto's is flexibility and personalization. Your dietary needs and preferences will be unique, and it's important to create a meal plan that aligns with your lifestyle and tastes. Here are a few tips to help you craft your own meal plan that supports thyroid health:

1. Focus on Whole, Nutrient-Dense Foods: Choose foods that are as close to their natural state as possible. Fresh vegetables, fruits, lean proteins, nuts, and healthy fats should be staples in your diet. These foods are rich in essential nutrients and free from the additives and preservatives found in processed foods.

2. Incorporate Anti-Inflammatory Ingredients: Include ingredients known for their anti-inflammatory properties, such as turmeric, ginger, garlic, leafy greens, berries, and fatty fish. These foods can help reduce inflammation, support immune function, and protect the thyroid gland.

3. Listen to Your Body: Pay attention to how your body responds to different foods. If you notice that certain foods trigger symptoms or make you feel unwell, consider eliminating them from your diet. Keeping a food journal can be helpful in identifying patterns and making adjustments as needed.

4. Stay Hydrated: Adequate hydration is essential for overall health and well-being. Water helps support digestion, circulation, and the elimination of toxins. Aim to drink at least eight glasses of water a day, and consider incorporating herbal teas and broths to add variety.

5. Plan Ahead: Meal planning and preparation can help ensure that you have healthy options available throughout the week. Consider batch cooking or preparing meals in advance to save time and reduce stress. This can also help you avoid reaching for less healthy options when you're in a hurry or feeling tired.

A Few More Recipes to Explore

Zucchini Noodles with Pesto and Grilled Shrimp: Spiralized zucchini noodles, or "zoodles," are a great alternative to traditional pasta. Toss them with a homemade pesto sauce made from fresh basil, garlic, olive oil, and pine nuts. Top with grilled shrimp for a protein-rich, low-carb meal that's bursting with flavor.

Rice and Roasted Vegetable Buddha Bowl: A Buddha bowl is a versatile meal that can be customized to include your favorite ingredients. Start with a base of rice, a complete protein rich in fiber and minerals. Add a variety of roasted vegetables, such as sweet potatoes, bell peppers, and broccoli, and top with a drizzle of tahini dressing and a sprinkle of sesame seeds.

Coconut and Lime Baked Cod: Cod is a mild, flaky white fish that pairs well with a variety of flavors. For a simple yet flavorful meal, marinate cod fillets in a mixture of coconut milk, lime juice, garlic, and cilantro, then bake until tender. Serve with a side of steamed asparagus or sautéed spinach for a light, refreshing dish.

Chia Seed Pudding: Chia seed pudding is an easy, make-ahead breakfast or snack that's rich in fiber and omega-3 fatty acids. Combine ¼ cup chia seeds with 1 cup unsweetened almond milk and 1 tablespoon maple syrup. Stir well and refrigerate overnight. In the morning, top with fresh berries, sliced almonds, and a drizzle of honey.

Embarking on a nutritional journey with Hashimoto's is about more than just following a set of rules or avoiding certain foods. It's about learning to nourish your body in a way that feels good, supports your health, and brings you joy. By experimenting with different recipes and meal plans, you can discover the foods that make you feel your best and create a sustainable, enjoyable approach to eating.

Remember that every person's needs are different, and what works for one individual may not work for another. Be patient with yourself as you explore different foods and cooking methods, and don't be afraid to make adjustments as needed. With time, practice, and a commitment to your health, you can develop a personalized diet that supports your thyroid, reduces symptoms, and enhances your overall well-being.

Conclusion

In this chapter, we have explored the profound impact that nutrition can have on managing Hashimoto's Thyroiditis. By focusing on essential nutrients such as iodine, selenium, zinc, and vitamin D, we can support thyroid health and modulate the immune system. At the same time, avoiding certain foods—like gluten, dairy, soy, and processed sugars—can help minimize inflammation and prevent symptoms from worsening.

The journey to finding the right dietary approach is deeply personal, requiring a willingness to experiment, listen to your body, and make adjustments based on your unique needs. Through mindful eating and thoughtful food choices, you can create a diet that not only supports your thyroid but also nourishes your entire body.

By incorporating the principles outlined in this chapter, you can craft a meal plan that aligns with your health goals and personal preferences. Remember, the path to managing Hashimoto's through nutrition is not about restriction, but rather about choosing foods that promote healing, reduce inflammation, and enhance overall well-being. With the right mindset and approach, you can use nutrition as a powerful tool in your journey toward optimal thyroid health and a vibrant life.

Lifestyle Modifications for Better Management

"The best project you will ever work on is yourself."

Managing Hashimoto's Thyroiditis is more than just a clinical process involving medications and regular check-ups; it's about embracing a holistic approach that encompasses all facets of daily life. Lifestyle modifications are a powerful tool in the arsenal for managing Hashimoto's. They go beyond treating symptoms and address the underlying factors that can either exacerbate or alleviate the condition. Research shows that a balanced lifestyle that includes appropriate exercise, effective stress management, and sufficient quality sleep can significantly improve the well-being of those living with Hashimoto's.

This chapter delves into the key lifestyle changes that can make a meaningful difference in managing Hashimoto's. We explore exercise programs specifically designed for individuals with this condition, focusing on the types of physical activity that promote strength and endurance without overwhelming the body. We also examine stress reduction techniques that can help calm the mind and body, reducing the inflammatory responses that can worsen symptoms. Finally, we discuss the importance of quality sleep and provide strategies to improve sleep hygiene and overall restfulness. By adopting these lifestyle modifications, you can create a more supportive environment for your thyroid health and enhance your overall quality of life.

6.1. Exercise Programs Suitable for Hashimoto's Patients

When it comes to individuals managing Hashimoto's Thyroiditis, exercise can have both positive and negative effects. Regular physical activity is a valuable tool for improving overall health, enhancing mood, and maintaining a healthy metabolism. However, if exercise is not approached with careful consideration, it can worsen fatigue, place additional stress on the body, and potentially contribute to burnout, particularly for individuals with already compromised energy levels. It is essential to select the appropriate exercise program for individuals with Hashimoto's. It's important to strike a balance between staying active and avoiding excessive strain on your body. The objective is to establish a sustainable exercise regimen that provides support to your body without exceeding its capabilities.

The Importance of a Customized Strategy

For individuals with Hashimoto's, it is crucial to adopt a personalized approach when it comes to exercise. Hashimoto's patients need to take into account various factors like thyroid hormone levels, adrenal health, and current symptoms when creating an exercise plan. The way you approach your actions, as well as the timing and frequency of those actions, are all important factors to consider. It is important to closely monitor your body's signals and be ready to make adjustments to your regimen as necessary.

Prior to embarking on a new exercise regimen, it is critical to seek guidance from your healthcare provider. They will evaluate your current health condition and identify any potential restrictions or factors to take into account. Performing blood tests to assess thyroid hormone levels, adrenal function, and overall fitness can offer valuable insights into determining the most suitable exercise regimen for you. Having a clear understanding of your overall health will enable you to prevent excessive strain and establish practical, attainable objectives.

Starting Slow: The Advantages of Low-Impact Exercise

Low-impact exercises can be a great option for individuals with Hashimoto's who are looking to gradually introduce physical activity into their daily routine. Engaging in low-impact exercises, such as walking, swimming, cycling, and yoga, can be beneficial for the joints and muscles, as they minimize the risk of injury or excessive strain. Engaging in these activities can have a positive impact on cardiovascular health, uplift mood, and aid in weight management, all while minimizing strain on the body.

Walking is a highly accessible and versatile form of low-impact exercise. Whether you're out for a casual stroll in your neighborhood or a more vigorous walk in the park, walking gives you the freedom to adjust your pace and intensity based on how much energy you have at the moment. Begin with shorter distances and gradually extend your duration as your endurance improves. Being surrounded by fresh air and natural scenery has its own set of advantages, including the potential to improve mental and emotional well-being by reducing stress and promoting a sense of overall wellness.

Swimming is a great choice for individuals with Hashimoto's. Immersing yourself in water can have a positive impact on your body, as it reduces stress on your joints and offers resistance to enhance your strength and endurance. Swimming can be especially helpful for those who are dealing with joint pain or stiffness. The warmth and buoyancy of the water can provide relief and enhance flexibility. Swimming is a calming and introspective activity that enables you to concentrate on your breath and movements, providing a release from stress.

Cycling, whether on a stationary bike or outdoors, provides a cardiovascular workout with minimal impact on your joints. It can be easily tailored to suit your fitness level. Cycling is a great way to enhance leg strength and boost cardiovascular health, all while minimizing stress on the knees and ankles. For outdoor enthusiasts, cycling offers a chance to discover new surroundings and savor the beauty of nature, leading to potential improvements in mental well-being.

Yoga is a wonderful exercise that combines physical movement, breath awareness, and mindfulness. It can be particularly beneficial for individuals who are managing Hashimoto's. The gentle stretching and strengthening postures contribute to enhanced flexibility, balance, and muscle tone, while the emphasis on deep, controlled breathing fosters a sense of relaxation and alleviates stress. Practicing yoga can provide significant advantages for those with Hashimoto's, as it focuses on enhancing both physical and mental well-being. This can lead to decreased fatigue, increased energy levels, and an overall improvement in one's state of health.

Building Strength: Incorporating Resistance Training

As you continue to enhance your energy levels and fitness, integrating resistance training into your exercise regimen can offer even more advantages. Resistance training utilizes various tools such as weights, resistance bands, or body weight to enhance muscle development and boost overall strength. Resistance training is beneficial for individuals with Hashimoto's as it can support metabolism, enhance bone density, and improve muscle tone. These factors play a crucial role in maintaining overall health and vitality.

When beginning a resistance training program, it is essential to prioritize correct form and technique to prevent any potential injuries. Start with lighter weights or resistance bands and incorporate exercises that focus on the major muscle groups, such as the legs, back, chest, arms, and core. It is recommended to schedule two to three sessions per week, ensuring adequate time for rest and recovery between workouts. As you gain more strength and confidence, you have the ability to gradually increase the weight or resistance and the number of repetitions.

By incorporating compound exercises like squats, lunges, push-ups, and rows, you can enhance the effectiveness of your workouts as they engage multiple muscle groups at once. Compound exercises are great because they imitate natural movements, which means they're functional and helpful for everyday activities. Always be attentive to your body's signals and make sure to modify the intensity and duration of your workouts according to your own sensations. It's advisable to begin at a moderate pace and steadily increase your strength rather than pushing yourself excessively and potentially facing injury or exhaustion.

Achieving Balance: The Importance of Flexibility and Mobility

Including flexibility and mobility exercises in your routine is helpful for maintaining overall health and preventing injury. Engaging in flexibility exercises, like stretching and yoga, can greatly enhance the range of motion in your joints and muscles. This, in turn, facilitates the execution of everyday tasks and minimizes the likelihood of experiencing strains and sprains.

Engaging in mobility exercises can greatly benefit individuals with Hashimoto's by targeting joint pain and stiffness, ultimately enhancing joint movement and function. Integrating dynamic stretches, foam rolling, and mobility drills into your warm-up and cool-down routines can contribute to the well-being of your joints and alleviate any discomfort.

An effective exercise program for individuals with Hashimoto's should encompass a variety of cardiovascular, strength, flexibility, and mobility exercises to promote overall well-being. Through a range of activities, you can boost your overall fitness, increase your energy levels, and minimize the impact of Hashimoto's symptoms on your daily routine.

Paying Attention to Your Body: The Significance of Rest and Recovery

Rest and recovery are critical components of an exercise program for individuals with Hashimoto's. Regular exercise is indeed beneficial, but it is equally important to allow your body sufficient time to recover and rebuild. Excessive training can result in heightened fatigue, muscle soreness, and potentially exacerbate symptoms of Hashimoto's.

Pay close attention to your body's signals and be mindful of how you feel before, during, and after physical activity. If you're experiencing fatigue or not feeling well, it's perfectly fine to give yourself a break or choose a more relaxing activity such as gentle yoga or a leisurely walk. Emphasizing the importance of rest and recovery will ensure that burnout is avoided and that your exercise routine remains sustainable in the long run.

By integrating techniques like stretching, foam rolling, and deep breathing exercises into your routine, you can enhance your recovery process. These methods work by alleviating muscle tension, inducing relaxation, and boosting circulation.

The Psychological Benefits of Exercise

Regular exercise can greatly improve mental and emotional well-being for individuals with Hashimoto's, in addition to its physical benefits. Research has demonstrated that regular physical activity can effectively alleviate symptoms of anxiety and depression, enhance mood, and promote optimal mental well-being. For individuals dealing with a chronic condition such as Hashimoto's, the psychological advantages of engaging in physical exercise can be just as significant as the physical ones.

Regular physical activity has numerous benefits, including boosting confidence, enhancing self-esteem, and cultivating a feeling of achievement. Engaging in physical activity can offer a beneficial means of managing stress and fostering social connections. This can be achieved through various avenues such as participating in group classes, team sports, or even taking a leisurely walk with a companion. By integrating regular exercise into your daily routine, you can establish a beneficial cycle that promotes your overall well-being, both physically and mentally.

For individuals with Hashimoto's, exercise goes beyond mere calorie burning or muscle building. It encompasses a comprehensive approach to health that nurtures the body, mind, and spirit. By selecting activities that bring you joy and are in line with your energy levels and objectives, you can establish a workout routine that improves your overall well-being.

It's important to keep in mind that your exercise program should be flexible and adaptable, allowing you to make adjustments based on your personal feelings and the needs of your body. Every individual has unique exercise needs, so it's crucial to discover the approach that suits you best. Through adopting a well-rounded and thoughtful approach to physical activity, you can effectively promote the health of your thyroid, alleviate symptoms, and enjoy a dynamic and energetic lifestyle while managing Hashimoto's.

Integrating exercise into your daily routine can be a game-changer when it comes to managing your health and optimizing your approach to Hashimoto's. By selecting activities that align with your unique requirements and prioritizing a comprehensive approach to wellness, you can make a significant difference in enhancing both your physical and mental well-being. As you delve into various exercise programs and discover the most suitable one for you, it's important to pay attention to your body, maintain patience with yourself, and acknowledge your achievements as you make progress.

6.2. Stress Reduction Techniques

Living with Hashimoto's Thyroiditis can be a difficult journey, often marked by unpredictability and varying symptoms. Stress, whether it's from physical strain or emotional turmoil, can worsen these symptoms, making it even harder to effectively manage them. Incorporating stress reduction techniques into your daily routine is absolutely critical for individuals with Hashimoto's. Managing stress involves more than just achieving a state of relaxation; it encompasses the reduction of inflammation, the balance of hormones, and the support of overall thyroid health. Creating a peaceful state of mind and a relaxed physical state can foster an internal atmosphere that supports healing and resilience.

Gaining Insight into the Effects of Stress on Hashimoto's

In order to fully grasp the significance of stress reduction, it is essential to have a comprehensive understanding of how stress impacts individuals with Hashimoto's. When stress strikes, the body's fight-or-flight response is activated, resulting in the release of stress hormones such as cortisol and adrenaline. When hormones are released in short bursts, they can be beneficial. However, if stress becomes chronic, these hormones can stay elevated and cause havoc on the body. Individuals with Hashimoto's may experience an intensified inflammatory response, compromised immune function, and hindered production of thyroid hormones due to prolonged stress.

During times of stress, the body focuses on essential survival functions rather than other processes such as digestion, immune regulation, and hormone balance. For individuals with Hashimoto's, whose thyroid function is already compromised, this can create a harmful cycle where stress further impairs thyroid function, resulting in worsening symptoms and heightened stress levels. Breaking this cycle is crucial, and one of the most powerful methods to achieve this is by practicing intentional stress reduction techniques.

The Benefits of Mindfulness and Meditation

Mindfulness and meditation are effective techniques for stress management and enhancing overall well-being. Practicing mindfulness entails being fully present in the current moment, free from any judgment. On the other hand, meditation is a technique that aims to train the mind to attain a state of tranquility and mental clarity. By following these practices, individuals with Hashimoto's can develop a sense of tranquility and embrace acceptance, even when faced with uncertainty and discomfort.

Regular mindfulness meditation has been shown to effectively reduce the body's stress response, lower cortisol levels, and foster a deep sense of relaxation. By reducing inflammation and supporting immune function, managing Hashimoto's becomes more feasible. Meditation can be simple and doesn't require a lot of time; just a few minutes each day can have a meaningful impact. Practicing simple techniques such as focusing on your breath, repeating a calming mantra, or visualizing a peaceful scene can effectively quiet the mind and alleviate stress.

If you're just starting out with meditation, guided meditation apps or online videos can be a great way to get started. These resources provide structured practices that will help you navigate each step, simplifying the process of getting started and establishing a routine. As you gain more experience with meditation, you can explore various techniques and discover which ones suit you the most.

Deep Breathing Exercises: An Easy and Powerful Technique

Deep breathing exercises are a straightforward and efficient method to decrease stress levels and encourage a state of relaxation. When we experience stress, our breathing often becomes shallow and rapid, indicating to our body that we are in a state of danger. By consciously slowing down and deepening our breath, we can send a calming signal to our body, indicating that it is in a safe state and enabling the parasympathetic nervous system to assume control. Activating this part of the nervous system can aid in stress reduction and promote healing, offering potential benefits for overall well-being.

An effective deep breathing technique is diaphragmatic breathing, also referred to as belly breathing. To practice this technique, find a cozy spot to sit or lie down and gently rest one hand on your chest while placing the other on your abdomen. Breathe in slowly through your nose, letting your belly expand while keeping your chest steady. Now, breathe out gently through your mouth, letting your stomach relax. Continue this practice for a few minutes, directing your attention to the feeling of your breath and releasing any stress or concern.

Another effective technique to try is the 4-7-8 breathing method. This involves inhaling for a count of four, holding the breath for a count of seven, and exhaling for a count of eight. This method is highly effective in promoting relaxation and alleviating feelings of anxiety, making it a valuable resource for stress management during the day or before going to sleep.

Progressive Muscle Relaxation for Stress Relief

Progressive muscle relaxation (PMR) is a method that entails deliberately tensing and subsequently releasing various muscle groups in the body in order to alleviate physical tension and encourage a state of relaxation. This practice can be especially helpful for individuals with Hashimoto's, as it aids in relieving muscle tension caused by stress and anxiety.

For effective PMR, it is important to locate a serene and cozy spot where you can either sit or recline. Begin by directing your attention to your feet and gradually contract the muscles, maintaining the tension for a brief period before releasing it as you exhale. Progress through the body, tightening and releasing every muscle group, from the calves and thighs to the abdomen, chest, arms, and face. As you continue, be mindful of the soothing feeling of relaxation that gradually envelops your entire body, enabling you to let go of any lingering tension completely.

Practicing PMR at any time can be beneficial, but it is particularly effective before going to bed as it helps to induce relaxation and enhance the quality of sleep. Similar to practices such as meditation and deep breathing, PMR is a straightforward technique that can be easily performed in any setting, making it a practical tool for effectively managing stress in everyday life.

The Incredible Healing Potential of Nature

Research has consistently demonstrated the multitude of advantages that spending time in nature can have on both mental and physical well-being. As a result, it has become widely recognized as an effective stress reduction technique, particularly for individuals with Hashimoto's. Being in nature has a soothing impact on both the mind and body, resulting in a decrease in stress hormones, a reduction in blood pressure, and the cultivation of a serene and contented state of being.

Engaging in outdoor activities such as strolling through a park, exploring the mountains, or peacefully sitting by a river can provide a much-needed respite from the pressures of everyday existence and allow for a reconnection with one's inner self.

Immersing oneself in the wonders of the natural world can offer a profound sense of tranquility and mental clarity.

For individuals residing in urban areas, discovering ways to integrate nature into their everyday lives can still yield substantial advantages. One option is to go for a stroll in a nearby park, another is to spend time tending to a garden, and you could also consider bringing plants into your home or workspace. It's important to take the time to pause, breathe, and fully embrace the beauty of the natural world, letting its soothing influence envelop you.

The Importance of Social Support and Connection

Having a strong support system and fostering connections with others are beneficial for effectively managing stress in individuals with Hashimoto's. Having a solid support system of loved ones and medical professionals can offer solace, motivation, and a feeling of connection, all of which are crucial for coping with stress and preserving mental well-being.

It can be incredibly valuable to connect with others who truly understand your experiences. Support groups, whether they are held in person or online, provide a valuable platform for individuals to connect, exchange personal stories, seek advice, and find solace among others who understand the challenges of living with Hashimoto's. These connections can foster a sense of community and alleviate the feelings of isolation that often accompany the management of a chronic condition.

It's important to have open and honest communication with your loved ones regarding your needs and boundaries. Inform them of ways they can provide support and clearly communicate your needs for effective stress and health management. Developing and nurturing meaningful connections can serve as a valuable shield against stress and establish a solid base of strength and adaptability.

Exploring Creative Activities for Stress Relief

Participating in artistic endeavors can be a potent method for alleviating stress and fostering emotional health. Engaging in creative activities such as painting, writing, playing music, or gardening can be incredibly fulfilling. These outlets allow you to express yourself, navigate your emotions, and experience pure bliss through the act of creation.

Discovering a creative outlet that speaks to you can offer a beneficial means of dealing with stress and effectively managing symptoms for those with Hashimoto's. Engaging in these activities can help you concentrate, get into a productive rhythm, and feel a deep sense of fulfillment and contentment. They can also serve as a welcome diversion from concerns and a means to direct your vitality towards something constructive and rewarding.

Ultimately, the most effective stress reduction techniques for managing Hashimoto's are the ones that best suit your personal preferences, lifestyle, and needs.

By integrating a range of stress reduction techniques into your daily routine, you can develop a holistic approach to managing Hashimoto's and promoting overall well-being. This comprehensive approach to stress management goes beyond simply reducing stress; it aims to cultivate a feeling of tranquility, strength, and self-empowerment in your daily life. With the proper tools and mindset, one can effectively navigate the challenges of Hashimoto's and cultivate a life that is harmonious, satisfying, and full of vitality.

6.3. Importance of Quality Sleep

Getting enough sleep is crucial for effectively managing Hashimoto's Thyroiditis. For individuals with this autoimmune disorder, sleep is not just a time of rest, but a vital period for the body to repair, restore, and regulate various systems, including the immune and endocrine systems. When sleep is disturbed or insufficient, it can have significant consequences, worsening symptoms, compromising immune function, and impeding the body's healing process. Recognizing the significance of getting good sleep and applying techniques to enhance it can have a significant impact on effectively managing Hashimoto's.

The Importance of Sleep for Thyroid Health

Sleep is essential for maintaining overall health, and its effects are especially significant for those with Hashimoto's. While we sleep, our bodies go through important processes that support immune regulation, hormonal balance, and cellular repair. Understanding these processes is important for effectively managing symptoms and avoiding additional complications in individuals with thyroid dysfunction.

Understanding the role of sleep in hormone regulation is crucial. Sleep plays a vital role in controlling the release of various hormones, such as thyroid hormones. The body's circadian rhythm, or internal clock, regulates the timing and release of these hormones, ensuring they are produced and secreted at optimal levels throughout the day. Insufficient sleep can throw off the body's natural rhythm, causing imbalances in thyroid hormone levels that may worsen symptoms like fatigue, weight gain, and mood disturbances.

In addition, sleep plays a vital role in supporting immune function. Sufficient sleep helps maintain a balanced immune response, which in turn helps to decrease inflammation and prevent the excessive immune activity commonly seen in autoimmune conditions such as Hashimoto's disease. On the other hand, lack of sleep can cause an increase in the production of pro-inflammatory cytokines, which can worsen the autoim-mune attack on the thyroid gland and make symptoms worse.

Exploring the Effects of Sleep Deprivation

Many people with Hashimoto's often struggle with sleep deprivation. Whether caused by the condition itself or external factors like stress, anxiety, or lifestyle habits, inadequate sleep can significantly impact overall health and well-being. Chronic lack of sleep can have negative effects on cognitive function, energy levels, and mental well-being, which can be particularly challenging for individuals with Hashimoto's.

Inadequate sleep can disturb the delicate equilibrium of hormones responsible for controlling hunger and metabolism, including leptin and ghrelin. This imbalance can result in heightened hunger and cravings, especially for foods rich in carbohydrates and sugars. This can contribute to weight gain and make it more challenging to manage Hashimoto's. The connection between sleep and metabolism works both ways: inadequate sleep can disrupt metabolic function, while metabolic problems can also impact the quality of sleep.

Understanding the impact of sleep deprivation is critical for individuals with Hashimoto's, as it helps prioritize sleep as a vital part of their management plan. Tackling sleep problems can play a huge role in disrupting the cycle of exhaustion, inflammation, and hormonal irregularities, leading to improved overall well-being.

Creating the perfect sleep environment

Establishing an ideal sleep environment contributes to enhancing the quality of sleep and fostering overall well-being. The bedroom should provide a peaceful environment for rest, free from any disturbances, and designed to promote relaxation. There are various factors that can contribute to creating the perfect sleep environment, such as temperature, lighting, noise levels, and overall comfort.

Temperature is a key factor when it comes to the quality of sleep. During sleep, the body's core temperature naturally decreases, and a cool room can assist in this process. It is generally recommended to maintain a bedroom temperature of 60-67 degrees Fahrenheit for optimal sleep. In addition, incorporating breathable bedding and opting for comfortable sleepwear can assist in maintaining a balanced body temperature and avoiding excessive heat during the night.

Exposure to light plays a crucial role in regulating the sleep-wake cycle. Getting enough natural light during the day, particularly in the morning, can strengthen your body's circadian rhythm and boost your alertness. On the other hand, being exposed to artificial light, especially blue light emitted from screens, during the evening hours can disrupt the natural production of melatonin. This hormone is responsible for signaling the body to get ready for sleep. For optimal sleep quality, it is recommended to reduce the brightness of lights in the evening and minimize screen usage before going to bed. Consider using blackout curtains or an eye mask to effectively eliminate any external light that could potentially disturb your sleep.

Noise can also affect the quality of sleep. While some individuals have no trouble sleeping through any noise, others may be more sensitive to their surroundings. Ensuring a peaceful setting is fundamental for undisturbed rest. If you find yourself easily bothered by noise, you might want to try using earplugs or a white noise machine to help drown out any disruptive sounds.

Getting a good night's sleep is vital for our well-being. Investing in a high-quality mattress and pillows that cater to your preferred sleep position can greatly enhance the quality of your sleep. Creating a sleep environment that is inviting and promotes relaxation can greatly improve your ability to fall asleep and stay asleep throughout the night.

Establishing a regular sleep routine

Establishing a regular sleep schedule can greatly enhance the quality of your sleep. Consistently maintaining a regular sleep schedule, including weekends, is crucial for maintaining a healthy sleep-wake cycle and regulating the body's internal clock. This regularity can contribute to a more restful sleep and a refreshed awakening.

Creating a soothing pre-sleep routine can effectively communicate to your body that it's time to relax and get ready for sleep, alongside maintaining a consistent sleep schedule. One possible routine could involve activities like reading a book, enjoying a warm bath, practicing gentle yoga or stretching, and engaging in relaxation techniques such as deep breathing or meditation. It's important to select activities that encourage relaxation and steer clear of stimulating activities like intense exercise, heated discussions, or consuming caffeine or alcohol in the evening.

Consistency plays a vital role in establishing a sleep routine. With some time and effort, your body can adapt to a new schedule and develop a healthier sleep pattern.

The Connection Between Nutrition and Sleep

Understanding the impact of nutrition on sleep quality is fundamental, as making conscious decisions about what we eat can greatly enhance our sleep. Some foods and nutrients have been found to support sleep, while others may disrupt it. For individuals with Hashimoto's, being mindful of their diet can have a positive impact on sleep quality and overall well-being.

Consuming foods that are abundant in tryptophan, an amino acid that the body converts into serotonin and melatonin, can be beneficial in promoting sleep. Turkey, chicken, eggs, nuts, seeds, and dairy products are excellent sources of tryptophan. In addition, including complex carbohydrates like whole grains, sweet potatoes, and legumes in your diet can enhance the availability of tryptophan in the brain, which can further promote better sleep.

However, the consumption of caffeine, sugar, and alcohol can have a negative impact on sleep patterns. Caffeine is a stimulant that can disrupt your ability to fall asleep and stay asleep, with its effects lasting for several hours. Avoiding caffeine in the afternoon and evening is recommended to minimize its impact on sleep. Consuming sugar can lead to changes in blood sugar levels that can disrupt sleep patterns, while alcohol may initially induce drowsiness but ultimately disrupt the sleep cycle and diminish the overall quality of sleep.

The Importance of Supplements in Promoting Healthy Sleep

For individuals with Hashimoto's who are experiencing sleep issues, supplements may provide some benefits. It's important to seek guidance from a healthcare professional prior to beginning any new supplement to ensure its safety and suitability for your individual requirements.

Magnesium is a mineral that contributes to more than 300 enzymatic reactions in the body, including those that promote relaxation and sleep. It plays a role in regulating neurotransmitters and melatonin, which helps control sleep-wake cycles. Adding magnesium supplements to your routine may contribute to a more relaxed state, alleviate muscle tension, and enhance the quality of your sleep, particularly if you have a deficiency.

Our bodies naturally produce melatonin in response to darkness. It plays a role in regulating the sleep-wake cycle and is commonly used as a supplement to promote better sleep, especially for those dealing with insomnia or jet lag. Using melatonin supplements can effectively signal to the body that it's time to sleep, facilitating the process of falling asleep and maintaining a restful sleep throughout the night.

Valerian root and passionflower are commonly used herbs known for their calming properties and ability to aid in sleep. These herbs are thought to possess properties that can soothe the nervous system, aiding in the reduction of anxiety and facilitating a peaceful sleep.

Supplements can certainly play a role in improving sleep, but it's important to remember that they should be just one piece of the puzzle. To truly manage sleep issues, it's important to adopt a holistic approach that encompasses lifestyle changes. This includes creating a sleep-friendly environment, establishing a consistent sleep routine, and incorporating stress reduction techniques.

It's important to keep in mind that getting enough sleep is essential for maintaining good health and overall well-being. Making sleep a top priority and incorporating it into your self-care routine can greatly enhance your ability to manage Hashimoto's and enhance your overall quality of life. By recognizing the significance of getting sufficient sleep and actively implementing strategies to promote it, you can establish a solid basis for improved well-being, endurance, and energy.

Conclusion

In this chapter, we have explored how important lifestyle modifications are for managing Hashimoto's Thyroiditis. Exercise, when chosen thoughtfully and performed regularly, can build strength, boost energy, and support overall health without putting undue stress on the body. By focusing on low-impact and moderate-intensity workouts, individuals with Hashimoto's can maintain an active lifestyle that enhances their physical and mental well-being.

We also discussed the importance of stress reduction techniques in managing Hashimoto's. Stress, both physical and emotional, can significantly impact thyroid health by exacerbating symptoms and triggering inflammatory responses. Incorporating mindfulness practices, deep breathing exercises, and other stress management strategies can help reduce the body's stress response and create a more balanced internal environment.

Quality sleep emerged as another critical component of effective Hashimoto's management. Restorative sleep is essential for hormone regulation, immune function, and overall health. By prioritizing sleep hygiene and creating an optimal sleep environment, individuals with Hashimoto's can enhance their ability to rest, recover, and manage their condition more effectively.

Together, these lifestyle modifications form a comprehensive approach to managing Hashimoto's that goes beyond medication and traditional treatments. By integrating these practices into your daily routine, you can take an active role in your health and well-being, fostering a more balanced, resilient, and vibrant life.

7

Advanced Care and Management

"The art of medicine consists of amusing the patient while nature cures the disease." — Voltaire

Managing Hashimoto's Thyroiditis often requires a multi-faceted approach that goes beyond conventional treatments. While thyroid hormone replacement therapy forms the foundation of management for many, a deeper understanding of the disease has paved the way for more advanced strategies. This chapter delves into the complexities of managing Hashimoto's beyond the basics, focusing on innovative treatments, navigating flares, and addressing the psychological impact of chronic illness. With over 14 million Americans affected by Hashimoto's, it is crucial to explore comprehensive strategies that not only alleviate symptoms but also enhance overall well-being.

In this chapter, we begin by exploring the latest innovations in treatment, from personalized medicine and genetic profiling

to biologic therapies and novel approaches like low-dose naltrexone. These advancements are not just about suppressing
symptoms but about targeting the underlying mechanisms
of the disease, offering new hope to those struggling with
persistent symptoms or complications. We also examine the
challenges of navigating flares and long-term complications,
providing practical advice on how to manage these unpredictable aspects of Hashimoto's. Finally, we address the
often-overlooked psychological impact of living with a chronic
illness, emphasizing the importance of mental health care and
resilience-building strategies. Together, these topics offer a
comprehensive overview of advanced care and management
for Hashimoto's, empowering patients to take control of their
health journey with confidence and optimism.

7.1. Navigating Flares and Long-Term Complications

Managing Hashimoto's Thyroiditis can be likened to a roller-
coaster ride, with its share of surprises, challenges, and setbacks along the way. Dealing with flares can be quite challenging for individuals living with Hashimoto's. These are
periods when symptoms suddenly worsen, often without any
clear reason. Alongside these unpredictable flares, people with
Hashimoto's may also experience long-term complications
that demand careful attention and proactive management.
Having a good grasp on how to overcome these obstacles is

essential for preserving well-being, reducing discomfort, and enhancing overall quality of life.

Understanding Hashimoto's Flares

Dealing with Hashimoto's flares can be incredibly frustrating and debilitating, as they bring about a sudden intensification of symptoms that can greatly disrupt your daily life. Typical symptoms experienced during a flare-up include profound fatigue, discomfort in the joints and muscles, cognitive difficulties, fluctuations in mood, and an overall feeling of unwellness. Flares of varying intensity and duration can occur, ranging from a few days to several weeks.

There are various factors that can potentially trigger a Hashimoto's flare-up. These factors can contribute to various health issues, such as stress, medication changes, infections, dietary indiscretions, or exposure to environmental toxins. Fluctuations in hormones, like the ones that happen during pregnancy, menstruation, or menopause, can also trigger a flare-up. For certain individuals, even seemingly minor alterations in their daily routine or lifestyle can result in a worsening of symptoms.

Although the precise mechanisms behind these flares remain somewhat elusive, they are believed to be associated with heightened autoimmune activity. In this scenario, the immune system erroneously targets the thyroid gland, resulting in inflammation and disturbances in the production of thyroid hormones. Being aware of the initial symptoms of a flare and taking immediate action can help minimize its effects and reduce its duration.

Strategies for effectively managing flares

Successfully managing a Hashimoto's flare necessitates a blend of personal awareness, proactive measures, and assistance from medical professionals. It is crucial to pay attention to your body and be aware of any early warning signs in order to effectively manage flares. Being aware of slight shifts in energy levels, mood, or physical symptoms can assist in recognizing the onset of a flare-up early on, enabling you to proactively mitigate its effects.

When experiencing a flare, it is essential to prioritize rest and self-care. It is important to minimize both physical and emotional stress since stress can intensify autoimmune activity and aggravate symptoms. It may be beneficial to consider taking a break from work, reducing your social commitments, and allowing yourself to rest. Engaging in gentle activities like yoga, meditation, and deep breathing exercises can effectively calm the mind and body, thereby reducing the intensity of the flare.

Proper nutrition is essential for effectively managing flares. When experiencing a flare, it is critical to prioritize the consumption of foods that have anti-inflammatory properties and are rich in nutrients. These types of foods can help boost immune function and alleviate inflammation. Proper hydration is crucial for maintaining optimal health and eliminating harmful toxins from the body. Eliminating known dietary triggers, such as gluten, dairy, and processed foods, can be beneficial in reducing irritation and inflammation.

Alongside making changes to your lifestyle, it may be necessary to collaborate closely with your healthcare provider in order to make adjustments to your medications or supplements during a flare-up. These steps may include a temporary increase in thyroid hormone replacement dosage, adjustments to other medications, or the addition of anti-inflammatory supplements. It is important to maintain regular communication with your healthcare team in order to effectively monitor symptoms and make any necessary adjustments to your treatment plan.

Managing Long-Term Complications

Managing flares is crucial for individuals with Hashimoto's, as it helps in maintaining a good quality of life. Additionally, it is essential to stay informed about potential long-term complications that may arise from this condition. These complications have the potential to impact multiple systems in the body and may necessitate continuous monitoring and management.

Hypothyroidism is a frequently observed long-term complication of Hashimoto's disease. It occurs when the thyroid gland fails to produce enough thyroid hormones. Hypothyroidism can cause a variety of symptoms such as fatigue, weight gain, sensitivity to cold, feelings of sadness, and difficulties with cognitive function. If hypothyroidism is not treated or managed properly, it can lead to significant health complications such as cardiovascular disease, infertility, and peripheral neuropathy.

For optimal management of hypothyroidism, it is crucial to maintain a close collaboration with your healthcare provider. This will ensure regular monitoring of your thyroid hormone levels and necessary adjustments to your medication dosage. It is essential to prioritize a healthy lifestyle, which involves maintaining a well-balanced diet, engaging in regular exercise, and effectively managing stress. These practices play a vital role in supporting thyroid function and promoting overall well-being.

Hashimoto's disease can potentially lead to the development of other autoimmune conditions. People diagnosed with Hashimoto's have a higher likelihood of developing additional autoimmune conditions, including type 1 diabetes, celiac disease, rheumatoid arthritis, or lupus. It is crucial to regularly screen for these conditions and remain vigilant for any new or worsening symptoms in order to detect and manage them early on.

Cardiovascular Health and Hashimoto's

Individuals with Hashimoto's, especially those with long-standing hypothyroidism, often have to pay close attention to their cardiovascular health. When the thyroid is underactive, it can cause a rise in cholesterol levels, an increase in blood pressure, and a greater susceptibility to atherosclerosis, which is the hardening of the arteries. These factors may heighten the likelihood of developing heart disease and stroke.

To effectively manage cardiovascular health, it is important to take a comprehensive approach. This involves regularly monitoring cholesterol levels, blood pressure, and other factors that contribute to cardiovascular risk. Making lifestyle changes, such as following a heart-healthy diet, staying physically active, and steering clear of smoking, is crucial in lowering the risk of cardiovascular problems. In certain situations, it may be necessary to consider the use of medications to help lower cholesterol or blood pressure. Collaborating with a knowledge-able cardiologist who specializes in handling cardiovascular problems related to the thyroid can offer valuable support and guidance.

Maintaining Bone Health with Hashimoto's

Individuals with Hashimoto's should also pay attention to their bone health. Insufficiently managed hypothyroidism may result in decreased bone density, elevating the chances of developing osteoporosis and experiencing fractures. This is particularly worrisome for postmenopausal women, who already face an increased vulnerability to bone loss.

Ensuring sufficient intake of calcium and vitamin D is crucial for maintaining strong bones and supporting bone health. Engaging in weight-bearing exercises like walking, jogging, or resistance training can effectively strengthen bones and lower the likelihood of developing osteoporosis. Regular bone density screenings may be advised for individuals at a higher risk, enabling early detection and intervention in case of bone loss.

Addressing Mental Health and Cognitive Function

It is crucial to not overlook the impact of Hashimoto's on mental health and cognitive function. People diagnosed with Hashimoto's disease have a higher likelihood of experiencing symptoms like depression, anxiety, and cognitive issues, including memory problems and trouble focusing. These challenges can become more pronounced during flares or when there is poor control over thyroid hormone levels.

Addressing mental health necessitates a holistic approach that encompasses both medical and psychological assistance. Consistently monitoring thyroid hormone levels and making necessary adjustments to medication can effectively alleviate cognitive and mood-related symptoms. Furthermore, reaching out to a mental health professional, like a therapist or counselor, can offer beneficial coping strategies and emotional support.

Participating in activities that enhance mental and emotional well-being, like mindfulness meditation, journaling, and quality time with loved ones, can also contribute to a better mood and cognitive function. Staying socially connected and engaging in activities that bring joy and fulfillment can offer a sense of purpose and help alleviate feelings of isolation.

A Comprehensive Approach to Managing Hashimoto's

Managing Hashimoto's requires a comprehensive approach that considers all aspects of health and well-being. This encompasses not just medical treatment, but also adjustments to one's lifestyle, assistance with emotional well-being, and prioritizing self-care. With a proactive and comprehensive approach to managing flares and long-term complications, you can enhance your quality of life and thrive with Hashimoto's.

Keep in mind that your experience with Hashimoto's is individual, and there isn't a universal solution for managing the condition. By staying well-informed, advocating for yourself, and embracing a comprehensive approach to care, you can successfully navigate the challenges of Hashimoto's with resilience, confidence, and optimism.

7.2. Innovations in Treatment

The treatment options for Hashimoto's Thyroiditis are constantly changing as medical research progresses and our understanding of autoimmune disorders deepens. With the advent of new technologies and advancements in our understanding of the disease, patients now have access to innovative treatments that offer renewed optimism in effectively managing their condition. These advancements go beyond traditional hormone replacement therapy, with a focus on tackling the root causes of Hashimoto's, alleviating symptoms, and enhancing overall quality of life. Through the exploration of these innovations, patients and healthcare providers can work together to develop tailored treatment plans that surpass traditional protocols.

Personalized Medicine and Genetic Profiling

Personalized medicine is a highly promising field of innovation in the treatment of Hashimoto's. This approach focuses on customizing medical treatment to suit the specific traits of each patient, taking into account factors such as their genetic makeup, lifestyle choices, and distinct biochemistry. Personalized medicine acknowledges the unique nature of each patient's experience with Hashimoto, which can be influenced by a range of genetic and environmental factors. Through a comprehensive understanding of these factors, healthcare providers can develop treatment plans that are more precise and impactful.

Understanding an individual's genetic makeup is critical in tailoring medical treatments to their specific needs. Thanks to recent advancements in genetic testing, it is now possible to pinpoint specific genetic variations that may make individuals more susceptible to autoimmune diseases such as Hashimoto's. For instance, specific genetic markers can suggest a greater chance of developing autoimmune thyroiditis or may uncover distinct patterns in immune system function that impact a patient's response to treatment.

Using this information, healthcare providers can customize interventions to suit the individual's genetic composition, selecting medications, supplements, and lifestyle adjustments that have the highest likelihood of success. Utilizing genetic profiling can aid in the identification of potential risks linked to specific treatments, enabling safer and more precise care. This individualized approach not only improves the effectiveness of treatment but also reduces the chances of negative side effects, making it a fundamental aspect of contemporary autoimmune care.

Biologic Therapies and Immune Modulation

Biologic therapies are a notable breakthrough in the management of Hashimoto's. These therapies utilize biologically derived molecules, like monoclonal antibodies, to specifically target components of the immune system. Biologics are specifically engineered to target the immune pathways responsible for autoimmune activity. By doing so, they effectively reduce inflammation and protect the thyroid gland from further damage, unlike traditional immunosuppressive drugs that have a broader impact on the immune response.

Research in this field is dedicated to the development of biologics that specifically target cytokines, which are essential signaling molecules involved in the immune response. In cases of Hashimoto's, there is an excessive production of specific cytokines, which results in the development of chronic inflammation and subsequent tissue damage. Through the inhibition of these cytokines, biologic therapies have the ability to regulate the immune system, thereby lessening the autoimmune assault on the thyroid and providing relief from symptoms.

Biologic therapy has shown promise in targeting B cells, which are a type of white blood cell responsible for producing antibodies. In autoimmune diseases such as Hashimoto's, B cells generate autoantibodies that target the body's tissues. Monoclonal antibodies that specifically target and deplete these B cells have demonstrated promising results in reducing autoantibody levels and alleviating symptoms in individuals with autoimmune thyroiditis. Biologic therapies are emerging as a promising option for treating Hashimoto's. These therapies aim to target the root cause of the condition by addressing the immune dysfunction, rather than just managing the symptoms.

Advancements in Thyroid Hormone Replacement

Thyroid hormone replacement continues to be the primary focus of Hashimoto's treatment, but there have been significant advancements that have resulted in more precise and efficient methods. Conventional hormone replacement usually includes the administration of levothyroxine. Nevertheless, not all patients exhibit optimal responses to T4-only therapy, and a subset of individuals still encounter symptoms even when their TSH levels are within the normal range.

Combination therapy with T4 and triiodothyronine (T3) has garnered significant attention as a potential solution to this problem. T3 is considered the more active form of thyroid hormone, and there are cases where patients may find it beneficial to use a combination of T4 and T3 in order to closely replicate natural thyroid function. With the development of sustained-release T3 formulations, it is now possible to maintain stable T3 levels throughout the day, minimizing the chances of experiencing symptoms due to fluctuations.

Exploring personalized dosing strategies is critical for optimizing hormone replacement, alongside combination therapy. Utilizing cutting-edge algorithms and genetic testing, we can accurately identify the optimal dosage and formulation for every individual. With a deep understanding of genetic variations in thyroid hormone metabolism and transport, healthcare providers can personalize hormone replacement to meet individual needs, resulting in enhanced symptom management and improved quality of life.

Low-Dose Naltrexone (LDN) and Other Innovative Treatments

Low-dose naltrexone (LDN) is a therapy that is gaining recognition for its potential benefits in autoimmune diseases, such as Hashimoto's. At lower doses, Naltrexone has been discovered to possess immune-modulating effects, although it is typically utilized in higher doses for treating opioid addiction. LDN is believed to function by temporarily inhibiting opioid receptors, resulting in a boost in the body's production of endorphins and other molecules that regulate the immune system.

LDN has shown promise in reducing inflammation and modulating the immune response for patients with Hashimoto's. This could potentially lead to a slowdown in the progression of the disease and an improvement in symptoms. Although the research on LDN for Hashimoto's is still in its early stages, there are promising indications from preliminary studies and anecdotal reports that it could be a beneficial additional treatment for certain patients.

Another area of research involves peptide therapy, where scientists are exploring the use of specific amino acid sequences to target immune pathways and potentially decrease inflammation. Peptide therapy aims to replicate the body's innate regulatory processes, providing a focused method for immune modulation. Stem cell therapy is also being extensively studied for its ability to regenerate damaged thyroid tissue and bring back normal thyroid function.

The Future of Hashimoto's Treatment

The future of Hashimoto's treatment is filled with exciting possibilities as research continues to advance. Novel treatments that focus on the fundamental causes of the illness, like immune modulation, provide renewed optimism for individuals striving to better control their condition. Advancements in medicine are allowing for more individualized and targeted interventions, while new treatments such as LDN and peptide therapy offer alternative ways to manage symptoms. Hormone replacement therapy and genetic profiling are also contributing to these exciting developments.

Ultimately, the aim of these advancements is to go beyond a generic approach to Hashimoto's treatment and towards a personalized, holistic strategy that caters to the specific requirements of every patient. By staying up-to-date on the latest advancements and collaborating closely with healthcare providers, patients can play an active role in their care and discover new possibilities for enhancing their health and quality of life.

The ever-changing field of Hashimoto's treatment demonstrates the impact of innovation and the significance of tailored care. With the emergence of new therapies, the management of Hashimoto's is becoming more effective, bringing renewed hope and a brighter future for individuals living with this chronic condition.

7.3. Psychological Impact of Chronic Illness

Living with Hashimoto's Thyroiditis, or any chronic illness, can be a difficult emotional journey. The chronic nature of the disease, along with its unpredictable symptoms and flares, can often have a profound psychological impact on individuals. For many individuals, dealing with Hashimoto involves not only physical challenges but also mental and emotional struggles. Having a deep understanding of the psychological impact of chronic illness is essential in order to develop a comprehensive approach to care that takes into account all aspects of a patient's well-being.

The Emotional Impact of Hashimoto's

Hashimoto's Thyroiditis is an autoimmune disorder that causes a wide range of symptoms that can fluctuate from day to day. Experiencing fatigue, weight gain, depression, anxiety, cognitive difficulties, and other symptoms can disrupt one's ability to carry out their daily activities. Such unpredictability often results in feelings of frustration, helplessness, and a sense of losing control, which can significantly impact mental well-being.

Depression is a prevalent issue among people diagnosed with Hashimoto's. Thyroid dysfunction can have a direct impact on mood and brain function, leading to feelings of sadness, hopelessness, and a lack of motivation. In addition, the fatigue and cognitive difficulties commonly faced by individuals with Hashimoto's can make it difficult to participate in activities that used to bring happiness, which can worsen symptoms of depression.

Living with a chronic illness often leads to anxiety, a common psychological response. The unpredictability of Hashimoto's disease can lead to a persistent sense of anxiety and apprehension, as one never knows when a flare-up might strike or how intense it might become. This anxiety can be heightened by worries about the future, such as the possibility of lasting complications and how the disease may affect one's work, relationships, and overall satisfaction in life.

Dealing with Chronic Illness: Discovering Inner Strength

Many individuals discover effective strategies to manage and develop resilience in the face of the overwhelming psychological impact of Hashimoto's. Resilience can be developed through a range of strategies and practices, enabling individuals to adapt and bounce back from challenging situations.

One of the best strategies for developing resilience is to prioritize what you have the power to influence, rather than fixating on what is beyond your control. One way to achieve overall well-being is by establishing a daily routine that incorporates activities promoting physical and mental health. This may include regular exercise, a nutritious diet, and sufficient rest. Creating a consistent schedule and organization can offer a sense of stability and predictability, which can be especially reassuring for individuals managing a long-term health condition.

Developing a positive mindset is a crucial component of building resilience. It is important to acknowledge the difficulties of living with Hashimoto and not to deny the reality of the situation. Instead, it requires finding strategies to shift one's perspective and concentrate on the positives, even when faced with challenging circumstances. Engaging in practices like gratitude journaling, mindfulness meditation, and cognitive behavioral therapy (CBT) can be beneficial in redirecting attention from negative thoughts to more constructive and empowering perspectives.

Having a strong network of friends and loved ones is essential for building resilience. Connecting with others who have similar experiences can offer a sense of validation, comfort, and camaraderie. Having a strong support system can greatly help in coping with the emotional effects of Hashimoto's. Whether it's through support groups, online communities, or loved ones, having people who offer understanding and encouragement can make a world of difference.

The Importance of Therapy and Counseling

Professional therapy or counseling can be extremely helpful for individuals with Hashimoto's in managing the emotional and psychological aspects of the disease. A qualified mental health professional can offer a secure and accepting environment to delve into emotions, navigate through feelings, and cultivate effective coping mechanisms.

CBT is a highly popular therapeutic approach for individuals dealing with chronic illness. CBT emphasizes the importance of recognizing and questioning negative thought patterns and replacing them with more balanced and realistic ones. This therapy can be especially beneficial for individuals with Hashimoto's who are facing challenges with depression or anxiety. It offers practical techniques to effectively manage these symptoms and enhance overall mental well-being.

ACT is a therapeutic approach that can offer potential benefits to individuals with Hashimoto's. ACT promotes the practice of embracing thoughts and feelings without passing judgment, while also taking actions that are in line with one's values and goals. This approach can assist individuals with Hashimoto's in discovering meaning and purpose, even when faced with difficult circumstances.

Alongside individual therapy, group therapy or support groups can offer a valuable sense of community and connection with others who are navigating similar challenges. Engaging in open conversations, empathizing with others, and providing encouragement can be a potent method to cultivate resilience and alleviate the sense of isolation.

The Influence of Long-Term Illness on Identity and Self-Concept

Living with a chronic illness such as Hashimoto's can have a profound effect on how a person perceives themselves and their identity. Many individuals with Hashimoto's often feel a profound sense of grief, as they grapple with the changes that come with the condition. They may mourn the loss of their previous identity, the abilities they once had, and the life they used to lead. These emotions can arise, causing a sense of loss, unhappiness, and a decrease in one's self-esteem.

Many people with Hashimoto's often grapple with their sense of self and may experience feelings of inadequacy or failure. The physical manifestations of the illness, including changes in weight, hair loss, and fatigue, can have a profound effect on one's self-esteem and body image, intensifying feelings of a diminished sense of self. In addition, the cognitive challenges commonly linked to Hashimoto's, such as difficulties with focus and memory, can pose obstacles in professional and personal spheres, resulting in feelings of frustration and self-questioning.

Reconstructing one's sense of identity and self-concept following a diagnosis of Hashimoto's requires discovering fresh ways to define oneself that go beyond the constraints imposed by the disease. One possible approach is to explore different interests, acquire new skills, or discover fresh ways to engage with the world. It is crucial to acknowledge and appreciate the strengths and qualities that persist, despite the challenges of illness. Discovering significance and direction in life, in spite of the obstacles posed by Hashimoto's, can assist individuals in cultivating a more optimistic and empowered sense of self.

Managing Relationships with Chronic Illness

Dealing with a chronic illness can deeply affect relationships, both internally and externally. Dealing with Hashimoto's can make it difficult to navigate relationships, as the disease often requires ongoing adjustments and accommodations that can impact interpersonal dynamics.

Effective communication is critical when it comes to managing relationships with chronic illness. Effective communication is crucial for fostering understanding and empathy among individuals with Hashimoto's and their loved ones. Sharing information about the disease, discussing its impact on daily life, and setting clear boundaries may be necessary. Sharing the difficulties of living with Hashimoto's can foster understanding and support from loved ones.

It is important for individuals with Hashimoto's to prioritize self-compassion and self-care within their relationships. It may be necessary to establish limits to safeguard one's energy and overall health, make self-care a top priority, and reach out for assistance when necessary. Seeking assistance and relying on the support of others is perfectly acceptable when facing challenging circumstances.

It's worth noting that chronic illness can actually foster stronger connections between individuals. Sharing the experience of living with Hashimoto can create stronger connections, cultivate empathy, and enhance relationships. Discovering ways to uplift each other, commemorate achievements, and overcome obstacles as a united front can foster a robust and unwavering support system.

Developing a Holistic Strategy for Mental Wellness

Addressing the psychological impact of Hashimoto necessitates a holistic approach that encompasses the various emotional, mental, and social difficulties linked to the condition. This could potentially include a mix of therapy, medication, adjustments to one's lifestyle, and the presence of a strong support system, all customized to meet the specific requirements and situations of each individual.

Alongside receiving professional support, incorporating self-care practices is essential for effectively managing the psychological impact of Hashimoto's. Participating in practices that encourage relaxation and alleviate stress, like meditation, yoga, or immersing oneself in nature, can effectively diminish stress levels and enhance overall well-being. Discovering methods to maintain an active lifestyle, consume a well-rounded diet, and ensure sufficient sleep can also contribute to the enhancement of mental and emotional well-being.

Ultimately, the aim of addressing the psychological effects of

Hashimoto's is to create a life that is purposeful, satisfying, and in line with one's personal values and aspirations. It's crucial to acknowledge that living with Hashimoto's is a continuous journey, with its fair share of highs and lows. With a proactive and comprehensive approach to care, individuals with Hashimoto's can cultivate resilience, discover joy, and live a fulfilling life, despite the obstacles of chronic illness.

Conclusion

As we conclude this chapter on advanced care and management for Hashimoto, it is clear that managing this condition requires a holistic and personalized approach. The journey of living with Hashimoto is not just about addressing physical symptoms but also about understanding and navigating the complexities of the disease. By exploring innovative treatments such as personalized medicine, biologic therapies, and novel interventions like low-dose naltrexone, patients and healthcare providers can work together to develop more effective, individualized care plans. These advancements provide new possibilities for managing Hashimoto's more effectively, reducing the burden of symptoms, and enhancing overall quality of life.

Navigating flares and long-term complications is another critical aspect of Hashimoto's management. Understanding the triggers and early signs of flares can help patients take proactive steps to minimize their impact, while addressing long-term complications requires ongoing monitoring and a comprehensive approach to care. The psychological impact of living with a chronic illness cannot be underestimated, and addressing mental health is an essential part of managing Hashimoto's. By building resilience, seeking support, and finding ways to cope with the emotional challenges of the disease, individuals can improve their well-being and maintain a positive outlook.

Ultimately, the goal of advanced care and management for Hashimoto's is to empower patients to live their best lives, despite the challenges of the disease. By staying informed, exploring new treatment options, and taking a proactive approach to both physical and mental health, individuals with Hashimoto's can navigate their journey with confidence, resilience, and hope for the future.

8

Beyond the Basics: The Role of Gut Health and Immunity

"All disease begins in the gut." — Hippocrates

This ancient wisdom has never been more relevant than it is today. Modern science is increasingly recognizing the profound connection between gut health and overall well-being, including the health of the thyroid and the immune system. For individuals with Hashimoto's Thyroiditis, understanding the role of gut health is not just an interesting tangent—it's essential. Researchers are discovering that the gut, often referred to as the "second brain," plays a crucial role in regulating immune function, inflammation, and even hormone production. This has significant implications for autoimmune diseases like Hashimoto's, where the immune system mistakenly targets the thyroid gland.

Studies have shown that individuals with autoimmune diseases, including Hashimoto's, often exhibit gut dysbiosis—an imbalance in the microbial communities living in the intestines. This imbalance can lead to increased intestinal permeability, also known as "leaky gut," which allows harmful substances to enter the bloodstream and trigger an inflammatory response that may worsen thyroid dysfunction. With over 70% of the immune system residing in the gut, it's clear that maintaining gut health is critical for keeping the immune system in check and reducing the autoimmune attack on the thyroid.

In this chapter, we'll go beyond the basics to explore how the gut influences thyroid health, immunity, and the body's ability to maintain balance. From understanding the gut-thyroid connection to exploring the benefits of probiotics, prebiotics, and ongoing research, this chapter will equip you with the knowledge to harness the power of gut health in your journey toward managing Hashimoto's and improving your overall well-being.

8.1. Understanding the Gut-Thyroid Connection

The saying that "all disease begins in the gut," originally credited to Hippocrates more than two millennia ago, has regained significance in contemporary medicine, especially when considering autoimmune conditions such as Hashimoto's Thyroiditis. Understanding the complex connection between the gut and the thyroid has become a topic of increasing interest, shedding light on how the well-being of the digestive system significantly affects thyroid function and overall immune health. In order to gain a comprehensive understanding of this correlation, it is necessary to explore the intricate ecosystem of the gut, the interconnections that tie it to thyroid well-being, and the ways in which promoting a healthy gut can aid in the management of Hashimoto's.

The Gut: A Pathway to the Immune System

The gut plays a vital role in not only digestion and nutrient absorption, but also in supporting the immune system. Around 70% of the immune cells in the body are located in the gut-associated lymphoid tissue (GALT), where they have continuous interactions with various microbes, food particles, and antigens. This interaction is crucial for the immune system to gain knowledge about what is harmless and what is potentially dangerous, allowing it to adjust its responses accordingly.

A well-functioning gut maintains a delicate equilibrium between immune tolerance and immune activation. Nevertheless, when the equilibrium is disturbed—due to various factors like unhealthy eating habits, high levels of stress, infections, or certain medications—the immune system may become imbalanced. This dysregulation can result in heightened intestinal permeability, often referred to as "leaky gut," where the integrity of the intestinal lining is compromised. When the intestinal barrier is compromised, larger, undigested food particles and toxins have the potential to enter the bloodstream, leading to an immune response that can cause inflammation throughout the body.

For people with Hashimoto's, this inflammation can worsen the autoimmune attack on the thyroid gland, resulting in additional harm and dysfunction. A strong correlation exists between the gut and the thyroid, with each influencing the other. A well-functioning gut promotes a healthy thyroid and balanced immune system, while a compromised gut can lead to thyroid issues and autoimmune disorders.

The Microbiome and Thyroid Health

The gut microbiome plays a crucial role in the connection between the gut and the thyroid. It consists of a diverse community of microorganisms, including bacteria, viruses, and fungi, that reside in the digestive tract. Understanding the microbiome's role in maintaining gut health, aiding in digestion, nutrient absorption, and the synthesis of essential vitamins and hormones is of utmost importance. It also plays a significant role in immune function, aiding in the regulation of the body's immune responses and reducing inflammation.

Studies have indicated that people with Hashimoto's disease frequently experience changes in their gut microbiome, including a decrease in diversity and an imbalance between beneficial and harmful bacteria. Such dysbiosis can potentially contribute to immune dysregulation and heightened intestinal permeability, thereby exacerbating inflammation and the risk of autoimmunity. Certain strains of bacteria have been found to have a significant impact on the conversion of inactive thyroid hormone (T4) to its active form (T3). This conversion is critical for proper thyroid function and metabolic regulation.

As an expert in the field, it is worth noting that the bacterial genus Bifidobacterium has been found to play a role in the conversion of T4 to T3. Additionally, certain bacteria like Lactobacillus contribute to the preservation of the intestinal lining and the prevention of leaky gut. When the population of these helpful bacteria is reduced, whether due to antibiotics, an unhealthy diet, or other factors, it disrupts the equilibrium of the microbiome. This disruption can have a chain reaction of consequences that negatively impact thyroid function and worsen autoimmune activity.

The Importance of Diet and Lifestyle in Maintaining Gut Health

Proper diet and lifestyle choices play a crucial role in main-taining optimal gut health, which in turn has a significant impact on the health of your thyroid. An unhealthy diet filled with processed foods, sugar, and unhealthy fats can lead to inflammation and throw off the balance of the gut microbiome. On the other hand, a diet that includes plenty of fiber, fermented foods, and nutrients with anti-inflammatory properties can help maintain a healthy gut environment.

Fiber, which can be obtained from a variety of sources such as fruits, vegetables, legumes, and whole grains, plays a vital role in maintaining a healthy gut. It supports the growth and activity of beneficial bacteria, enhancing their overall function. This process, referred to as fermentation, results in the production of short-chain fatty acids (SCFAs) like butyrate. These SCFAs possess anti-inflammatory properties and contribute to the preservation of the intestinal lining's integrity. Through the promotion of a healthy gut microbiome and the maintenance of intestinal well-being, a diet rich in fiber can aid in the reduction of inflammation and the maintenance of immune balance, both of which play a vital role in the management of Hashimoto's.

Fermented foods like yogurt, kefir, sauerkraut, and kimchi help maintain a gut-friendly diet. These foods have live beneficial bacteria, or probiotics, which can aid in replenishing and diversifying the gut microbiome. Consuming fermented foods regularly has been proven to have positive effects on gut health, immune function, and inflammation reduction. This makes them beneficial in the management of autoimmune diseases such as Hashimoto's.

Aside from diet, lifestyle factors like stress, sleep, and physical activity also have a major impact on gut health. Chronic stress has the potential to impact the gut microbiome, leading to changes in its composition. This, in turn, can result in increased intestinal permeability and inflammation, which may worsen autoimmune activity. Practicing mindfulness, meditation, and engaging in regular exercise can be beneficial for maintaining gut health and minimizing the effects of stress on the immune system.

Sufficient sleep is essential for maintaining a healthy gut, as the gut microbiome is regulated by the body's sleep-wake cycle. Sleep disturbances can have a significant impact on the gut microbiome, leading to immune dysregulation and increased inflammation. Emphasizing the importance of getting sufficient sleep is critical for promoting gut health and effectively managing Hashimoto's.

The Influence of Medications on Gut Health

Certain medications, such as antibiotics, nonsteroidal anti-inflammatory drugs (NSAIDs), and proton pump inhibitors (PPIs), can greatly affect the health of your gut. Although antibiotics are essential for treating infections, they can disturb the delicate equilibrium of the gut microbiome by eliminating both harmful and beneficial bacteria. This disturbance can result in an imbalance of gut bacteria and heightened permeability of the intestines, which can contribute to inflammation and the activation of the immune system.

Nonsteroidal anti-inflammatory drugs (NSAIDs), which are frequently prescribed for pain management and reducing inflammation, have the potential to harm the lining of the intestines and raise the likelihood of developing leaky gut. It's important to note that PPIs, commonly used to treat acid reflux and heartburn, have the potential to impact the balance of the gut microbiome and decrease the production of stomach acid, which plays a big role in digestion and absorbing nutrients. It is important to use these medications cautiously and consider alternative treatments whenever feasible, as their prolonged use may lead to gut dysbiosis and compromised immune function.

It is critical for those with Hashimoto's to understand the potential effects of medications on gut health and collaborate with healthcare professionals to reduce their usage whenever feasible. It may be worth considering alternative treatments, like natural anti-inflammatories or digestive support supplements, which have a reduced chance of affecting the gut microbiome and causing inflammation.

Healing the Gut to Support Thyroid Health

Understanding the significant link between gut health and thyroid function, it becomes evident that addressing gut health is an essential aspect of effectively managing Hashimoto's. This process focuses on identifying and resolving the root causes of gut dysfunction, including dysbiosis, leaky gut, and inflammation. It also involves implementing strategies to promote balance and enhance gut health.

Identifying and eliminating potential triggers of inflammation and dysbiosis is crucial in the healing process of the gut. Working alongside a healthcare provider, it may be necessary to identify potential food sensitivities, such as gluten or dairy, that can cause irritation to the gut lining and contribute to inflammation. Following an elimination diet can be beneficial in pinpointing specific triggers and guiding necessary dietary adjustments. This involves temporarily eliminating common inflammatory foods from your diet and gradually reintroducing them one by one.

Aside from making adjustments to your diet, incorporating specific supplements can also contribute to improving gut health. Probiotics, with their beneficial bacteria, help rebalance the gut microbiome and bolster immune function. Prebiotics, being non-digestible fibers that act as nourishment for beneficial bacteria, play a crucial role in enhancing the growth and function of these bacteria, thus contributing to the well-being of the gut.

Additional supplements that could potentially support gut healing are digestive enzymes, which assist in the breakdown and absorption of nutrients, and glutamine, an amino acid that promotes the integrity of the intestinal lining. Omega-3 fatty acids, known for their anti-inflammatory properties, can contribute to reducing inflammation and promoting gut health.

It is crucial to prioritize lifestyle modifications, including stress management, sufficient sleep, and consistent physical activity, to effectively support gut health. By considering these factors and adopting a holistic approach to gut healing, individuals with Hashimoto's can effectively promote their thyroid health and minimize the effects of autoimmune activity.

Having a deep understanding of the gut-thyroid connection is vital when it comes to developing a holistic approach to effectively managing Hashimoto's. The gut and the thyroid have a close relationship, with each impacting the function and balance of the other. By focusing on gut health and addressing the root causes of gut dysfunction, individuals with Hashimoto's can enhance their thyroid health, decrease inflammation, and enhance their overall well-being.

8.2. Probiotics and Prebiotics

When it comes to achieving optimal health, particularly in the management of conditions such as Hashimoto's Thyroiditis, the importance of gut health cannot be emphasized enough. Probiotics and prebiotics play a vital role in promoting a healthy gut. These two components work in harmony to support the gut microbiome, which in turn enhances immune function and thyroid health. Gaining a thorough understanding of how these elements operate, the advantages they offer, and how to seamlessly integrate them into your daily routine can have a profound impact on managing autoimmune conditions and fostering overall holistic well-being.

Probiotics: The Beneficial Bacteria

Probiotics are live microorganisms, commonly known as "good" or "friendly" bacteria, that provide health benefits when consumed in sufficient quantities. These helpful bacteria contribute to the maintenance of a balanced gut microbiome, a complex community of microorganisms that supports digestion, nutrient absorption, and immune regulation. Supporting a healthy and balanced gut microbiome is crucial in the context of Hashimoto's, where immune system dysregulation is a core issue.

Probiotics function by establishing a presence in the gut and engaging in healthy competition with detrimental bacteria for both space and resources. They create substances that hinder the growth of harmful microbes, strengthen the gut lining, and promote the production of compounds that regulate the immune system. Some strains of probiotics, like Lactobacillus and Bifidobacterium, are highly effective in regulating immune responses, decreasing inflammation, and supporting a harmonious gut bacteria ecosystem. These strains have been found to contribute to the reduction of intestinal permeability commonly associated with "leaky gut," a condition that can worsen autoimmune activity.

For those with Hashimoto's, adding probiotics to your diet can provide relief from symptoms, enhance digestion, and boost your immune system. Probiotics can be acquired through various means, including both food and supplements. Fermented foods, in particular, are highly regarded as an excellent source of these beneficial microorganisms. Yogurt, kefir, sauerkraut, kimchi, miso, and tempeh are excellent sources of live cultures that can nourish and enhance the gut microbiome. When selecting probiotic-rich foods, it's crucial to opt for raw and unpasteurized options since pasteurization can eliminate the helpful bacteria.

Probiotic supplements are a great option to maintain a consistent and sufficient intake of beneficial bacteria, alongside fermented foods. When choosing a probiotic supplement, it's crucial to opt for one that includes a range of strains, such as Lactobacillus and Bifidobacterium. Additionally, it's essential to select a formulation that can withstand the acidic conditions of the stomach, allowing the bacteria to reach the intestines where they can provide their advantageous effects. Consulting with a healthcare provider can help determine the most appropriate product and regimen for individual needs, as dosage and strain diversity play a crucial role in the effectiveness of probiotic supplements.

Prebiotics: Feeding the Microbiome

Probiotics work by introducing beneficial bacteria into the gut, while prebiotics act as the nourishment that fuels the growth and activity of these bacteria. Prebiotics are a form of non-digestible fiber that moves through the upper portion of the gastrointestinal tract without being broken down by digestive enzymes. Instead, they make their way to the colon, where they undergo fermentation by the gut microbiota. This process results in the production of short-chain fatty acids (SCFAs), which offer significant health advantages.

Some of the most commonly used prebiotics are inulin, fructooli gosaccharides (FOS), galactooligosaccharides (GOS), and resistant starches. These fibers can be found in a range of plant-based foods, such as onions, garlic, leeks, asparagus, bananas, oats, and Jerusalem artichokes. By regularly incorporating these foods into your diet, you can promote a healthy gut environment, leading to improved gut health, reduced inflammation, and enhanced immune function.

Gut bacteria produce short-chain fatty acids (SCFAs), including butyrate, acetate, and propionate, through the fermentation of prebiotics. These short-chain fatty acids have numerous important functions in maintaining gut health. They provide energy for colon cells, enhance the integrity of the gut barrier, decrease inflammation, and contribute to the regulation of immune function. Research has demonstrated that butyrate possesses anti-inflammatory properties and supports the health of the intestinal lining, making it crucial for preventing and managing leaky gut.

For individuals with Hashimoto's, it is key to maintain a diet that is abundant in prebiotic fibers. This is because prebiotic fibers play a vital role in supporting the gut microbiome, which in turn contributes to maintaining optimal thyroid health. It is critical to gradually introduce prebiotics, particularly if you have a sensitive digestive system. This is because a sudden increase in fiber intake can cause bloating and discomfort. Beginning with small quantities and gradually increasing consumption enables the digestive system to adjust and may assist in reducing any negative consequences.

The Power of Probiotics and Prebiotics Working Together

The connection between probiotics and prebiotics is mutually beneficial, as they collaborate to enhance gut health. Probiotics require prebiotics to flourish, while prebiotics depend on probiotics to ferment them into advantageous compounds such as SCFAs. This harmonious connection is often called synbiotics, which refers to products or routines that combine probiotics and prebiotics to optimize their health advantages.

Including both probiotics and prebiotics in your diet can greatly improve the health of your gut microbiome, boosting its diversity and resilience. These factors can contribute to enhanced digestion, increased nutrient absorption, and a more harmonized immune response, all of which play a crucial role in managing Hashimoto's. Combining probiotic-rich foods or supplements with prebiotic-rich foods can greatly enhance gut health and contribute to overall well-being.

For instance, combining a bowl of yogurt that is rich in probiotics with oats or bananas that are rich in prebiotics can result in a well-rounded meal that promotes a healthy gut microbiome. A salad crafted with fresh garlic, onions, and asparagus, complemented by a tangy dressing such as kimchi or sauerkraut, offers a powerful blend of probiotics and prebiotics that collaborate to support and fortify the gut.

Customizing Probiotic and Prebiotic Consumption to Suit Personal Requirements

Although probiotics and prebiotics have numerous advantages for gut health, it's important to acknowledge that everyone's requirements may differ. Various factors, including gut sensitivity, existing health conditions, and dietary preferences, contribute to determining the most suitable approach to probiotic and prebiotic intake.

Certain probiotic strains may provide greater benefits for certain individuals. For instance, individuals who have previously taken antibiotics or experienced frequent infections might find it advantageous to consume more strains of Lactobacillus and Bifidobacterium. These particular strains are recognized for their ability to support the immune system. Individuals with certain gut health concerns, like irritable bowel syndrome (IBS), might experience relief from strains such as Saccharomyces boulardii or Bacillus coagulans. These strains have demonstrated the ability to promote digestive function and alleviate symptoms.

It is important to customize the selection of prebiotics based on individual tolerance levels. Certain individuals may have a higher sensitivity to specific types of fiber, like inulin, which can lead to bloating or discomfort when consumed in excessive quantities. When faced with such situations, it may be more comfortable to begin with smaller quantities or opt for different sources of prebiotics, such as resistant starches found in cooked and cooled potatoes or green bananas, to promote gut health.

Collaborating with a healthcare provider or a nutritionist can assist in customizing a probiotic and prebiotic regimen that is most suitable for your specific requirements. This tailored approach guarantees that you receive the optimal combination of helpful bacteria and the essential nutrients they require to flourish, all while minimizing any possible discomfort or negative consequences.

Exploring the Systemic Benefits of Probiotics and Prebiotics

The advantages of probiotics and prebiotics go well beyond the digestive system. Through their impact on the gut microbiome, these components can have far-reaching effects on various aspects of well-being, such as the immune system, mental well-being, and even the health of the skin. Research has shown that there is a strong connection between gut health and mental well-being. The gut-brain axis, in particular, emphasizes this link. Recent studies have indicated that maintaining a healthy microbiome can have positive effects on mood, cognitive function, and stress resilience.

For people with Hashimoto's, the systemic advantages of probiotics and prebiotics are especially significant. Through the reduction of inflammation, support for immune balance, and improvement of gut health, these components have the potential to effectively manage the symptoms of Hashimoto's and enhance overall well-being. Incorporating probiotics and prebiotics into your daily routine can be a game-changer for your health, helping your body heal and thrive naturally. Whether you choose to get them from food or supplements, these powerful strategies can give you more control over your well-being.

Ultimately, probiotics and prebiotics play a crucial role in effectively managing Hashimoto's Thyroiditis and promoting optimal gut health. By gaining a deep understanding of their roles, selecting the appropriate sources, and customizing your intake to meet your specific needs, you can fully utilize their capabilities to promote a thriving gut microbiome, boost immune function, and enhance your overall state of well-being. With ongoing research, the significance of these gut-friendly components becomes increasingly evident, providing a route to improved health through the influence of nutrition and microbiome support.

8.3. Ongoing Research and What It Means for You

Over the past few years, the scientific community has shown great interest in studying the relationship between gut health, immunity, and thyroid function. Scientists globally are extensively studying the intricate connections between these systems, uncovering fresh perspectives that have the potential to revolutionize the treatment of Hashimoto's Thyroiditis and other autoimmune conditions. Staying informed about these ongoing studies is not only interesting, but also empowering for individuals living with Hashimoto's. The results of these studies have the potential to greatly influence future treatment approaches and provide innovative strategies for more efficient management of the condition. Within this subchapter, we will delve into the most encouraging realms of ongoing research and their implications for you.

Exploring the Gut-Brain-Thyroid Axis

The gut-brain axis, which involves the communication network between the gut and the brain, is widely recognized and understood. Recent research is broadening the scope of this concept to encompass the thyroid, resulting in the emergence of the gut-brain-thyroid axis. In this fascinating area of research, scientists are delving into the intricate connections between the gut microbiome, brain function, and thyroid activity.

Stress, for instance, has been found to impact both gut health and thyroid function. Chronic stress has the potential to disturb the equilibrium of the gut microbiome, resulting in dysbiosis and heightened intestinal permeability. Consequently, this can potentially initiate or exacerbate autoimmune thyroid conditions. On the other hand, when there is an issue with the thyroid, it can have an impact on mood and cognitive function, creating a cycle that affects overall well-being.

Current research is exploring the potential benefits of interventions that focus on the connection between the gut, brain, and thyroid in individuals with Hashimoto's, aiming to improve their outcomes. I am well-versed in various approaches to improve gut health, reduce inflammation, and optimize thyroid function. This involves investigating the potential benefits of probiotics, prebiotics, dietary modifications, and stress management techniques. Having a deep understanding of these intricate interactions could pave the way for more holistic approaches to effectively managing Hashimoto's, taking into account both the physical and psychological dimensions of the condition.

Exploring the Potential of Immune Modulation Therapies

Ongoing research is focused on finding innovative approaches to optimize immune responses and enhance the well-being of patients. I am particularly interested in the development of biologic therapies, which are drugs derived from living organisms that specifically target components of the immune system.

When it comes to Hashimoto's, there are biologics available that specifically target cytokines, which are proteins responsible for immune signaling. These biologics have the potential to reduce inflammation and protect the thyroid gland from the immune system's attacks. As an expert in the field, I can provide an example of how researchers are studying monoclonal antibodies that can block the action of certain cytokines, like tumor necrosis factor (TNF) or interleukin-6 (IL-6), to potentially regulate immune responses in autoimmune thyroiditis.

Another area of research that shows promise is the utilization of low-dose naltrexone (LDN), a medication typically prescribed for opioid addiction. At lower doses, naltrexone has demonstrated the ability to regulate immune function by boosting the production of endorphins. This, in turn, can promote immune regulation and alleviate inflammation. Initial research indicates that LDN might offer potential benefits in alleviating symptoms and enhancing the overall well-being of individuals with autoimmune conditions, such as Hashimoto's.

As these therapies are further researched, they have the potential to provide innovative, focused treatments for Hashimoto's that surpass conventional hormone replacement therapy. These treatments aim to target the root cause of the disease, which is immune dysregulation.

The Future of Hashimoto's Research

The field of Hashimoto's research is constantly evolving, with new discoveries and advancements emerging at a remarkable pace. Researchers are making groundbreaking discoveries in the field of autoimmune thyroid diseases, delving into the gut microbiome's influence on immune function and developing personalized nutrition plans and targeted therapies. These findings have the potential to completely transform our understanding and management of these conditions.

Staying informed about ongoing research is crucial for individuals with Hashimoto's, as it is a proactive measure towards improving their health. With a deep understanding of the most recent research and its potential impact, individuals can have meaningful conversations with their healthcare providers, discover innovative treatment choices, and confidently take charge of their own healthcare.

In the coming years, the field of Hashimoto's research shows great potential for developing individualized, efficient, and comprehensive methods to effectively manage the condition. With the expanding knowledge of the intricate connections between the gut, immune system, and thyroid, new treatment options are emerging that hold promise for individuals with Hashimoto's, providing them with hope and potential healing.

9

Conclusion

Final Thoughts and Encouragement for the Journey Ahead

As you reach the end of this book, it's important to take a moment to reflect on the journey you've embarked upon in understanding and managing Hashimoto's Thyroiditis. Navigating a chronic illness is rarely straightforward; it's filled with ups and downs, victories and setbacks, moments of clarity, and times of doubt. But through it all, what truly matters is your commitment to taking control of your health, to learning, adapting, and persevering. This book has been a guide to understanding the complexities of Hashimoto's and providing you with the tools and strategies to manage it effectively. But beyond these pages lies the real essence of your journey—your own personal story of resilience, strength, and hope.

Living with Hashimoto's, or any chronic condition, can feel

overwhelming at times. It can be frustrating to deal with symptoms that fluctuate, making each day unpredictable. You may find yourself longing for the days when you didn't have to think about every meal, every supplement, every ounce of energy spent. It's normal to feel this way. It's normal to wish for a simpler path. But in these moments of frustration and fatigue, remember that every step you take towards understanding and managing your condition is a step towards reclaiming your life.

What you've learned here is just the beginning. You now have a foundation of knowledge about how Hashimoto affects the body, the importance of diet, the role of the gut, and the myriad ways you can support your thyroid health through lifestyle changes and medical interventions. Armed with this information, you are better equipped to make informed decisions, advocate for yourself, and seek out the care and support you need. Knowledge is power, but the real power comes from applying that knowledge in your daily life, in making choices that support your well-being and in embracing the idea that you have more control over your health than you might have once believed.

There will be days when it feels like you're moving forward and days when it feels like you're taking two steps back. This is part of the journey. Health is not a destination but a continuous process of learning, adapting, and growing. You are not alone in this experience. Countless others are walking a similar path, facing the same challenges, and finding ways to thrive despite the obstacles. Community and connection can be powerful allies. Reach out, share your story, listen to others, and find strength in the shared experience of those who understand what you're going through.

Self-compassion is another crucial companion on this journey. It's easy to be hard on yourself, to feel like you're not doing enough or that you're not doing things right. But remember, perfection is not the goal. Progress is. Small steps, small changes, and small victories all add up over time. Celebrate them. Celebrate yourself for showing up, for trying, for caring about your health and well-being. Self-compassion means treating yourself with the same kindness and understanding you would offer a friend. It means acknowledging your efforts, forgiving your missteps, and giving yourself permission to rest when needed.

As you move forward, keep exploring and experimenting with what works best for you. Health is deeply personal, and what works for one person may not work for another. Listen to your body. It has a wisdom all its own. Pay attention to how different foods, activities, and treatments make you feel. Keep a journal if it helps, track your symptoms, your energy levels, your mood. Over time, patterns will emerge, and you'll gain a clearer understanding of what supports your health and what doesn't. This process of self-discovery is invaluable. It empowers you to take charge of your health in a way that no one else can.

Stay curious and stay open. Science and medicine are continually evolving fields. New research, new treatments, and new insights are always on the horizon. Stay informed about the latest developments in thyroid health, autoimmune conditions, and integrative medicine. Be open to new ideas and approaches, but also trust your instincts. You are the expert on your own body, and you have the right to decide what feels right for you.

Remember, too, the importance of balance. Managing Hashimoto's is important, but so is living your life. Don't let the condition define you or limit your experiences. Make time for the things that bring you joy, that nourish your soul, and that make you feel alive. Whether it's spending time with loved ones, pursuing a passion, traveling, or simply enjoying a quiet moment in nature, these experiences are just as vital to your health as any diet or supplement.

There will be times when you need to push yourself, and there will be times when you need to rest. Learning to recognize these moments and honor them is a crucial part of the healing process. It's about finding that delicate balance between effort and ease, between striving for better health and accepting where you are right now.

As you continue on your path, know that it's okay to seek help. Whether it's from a healthcare provider, a nutritionist, a therapist, or a friend, asking for support is a sign of strength, not weakness. You don't have to do this alone. There are many resources and communities out there dedicated to helping people with Hashimoto's. Find the ones that resonate with you and lean on them when you need to.

Finally, never underestimate the power of hope. Hope is a driving force that keeps us moving forward, even when the path is unclear. Hope is not about expecting that everything will always be perfect or that there will never be challenges. It's about believing in the possibility of better days, of healing, and of a life lived fully and richly, regardless of the circumstances. Hope is what allows us to dream, to set goals, and to pursue them with passion and determination.

As you close this book, take a deep breath and remind yourself of how far you've come. The journey with Hashimoto's is not an easy one, but it is one that you are navigating with courage, resilience, and grace. Continue to be kind to yourself, continue to advocate for your health, and continue to seek out the knowledge and support that empowers you to live your best life.

Your journey is uniquely yours, and it is filled with opportunities for growth, learning, and transformation. Embrace it. Trust it. And know that with every step you take, you are moving closer to a place of greater health, balance, and well-being. The road ahead may be long, but it is also full of possibilities.

Here's to the journey ahead—may it be one of hope, healing, and endless discovery.

Afterword

Glossary of Key Terms

1. Autoimmune Disease: A condition in which the immune system mistakenly attacks the body's own tissues, considering them foreign invaders. In the case of Hashimoto's Thyroiditis, the immune system targets the thyroid gland.
2. Hashimoto's Thyroiditis: An autoimmune disorder characterized by chronic inflammation of the thyroid gland, leading to hypothyroidism. It is the most common cause of hypothyroidism in the United States.
3. Hypothyroidism: A condition where the thyroid gland does not produce enough thyroid hormones, leading to symptoms such as fatigue, weight gain, and depression.
4. Thyroid Gland: A butterfly-shaped gland located in the front of the neck that produces hormones regulating metabolism, heart rate, and body temperature.
5. Thyroid Hormones: Hormones produced by the thyroid gland, primarily thyroxine (T4) and triiodothyronine (T3), which are crucial for metabolism, growth, and development.
6. Leaky Gut: A condition characterized by increased intestinal permeability, where the gut lining becomes compro-

mised, allowing undigested food particles, toxins, and microbes to enter the bloodstream, potentially triggering immune responses.

7. Microbiome: The community of microorganisms, including bacteria, viruses, fungi, and other microbes, that inhabit various parts of the body, especially the gut, and play a significant role in health and disease.

8. Probiotics: Live microorganisms, often referred to as "good" or "friendly" bacteria, that provide health benefits when consumed, particularly for digestive and immune health.

9. Prebiotics: Non-digestible fibers that serve as food for beneficial bacteria in the gut, promoting their growth and activity.

10. Short-Chain Fatty Acids (SCFAs): Byproducts of the fermentation of dietary fibers by gut bacteria. SCFAs, such as butyrate, acetate, and propionate, play a critical role in gut health and immune regulation.

11. Biologic Therapies: Treatments derived from living organisms or their products, used to target specific components of the immune system in autoimmune diseases.

12. Low-Dose Naltrexone (LDN): A medication used at low doses to modulate immune function and reduce inflammation in autoimmune conditions.

13. Personalized Nutrition: A tailored approach to diet that considers an individual's unique genetic makeup, microbiome composition, and metabolic profile to optimize health outcomes.

14. Gut-Brain Axis: The bidirectional communication network between the gut and the brain, highlighting the connection between digestive health and mental well-

being.

15. Immune Modulation: The process of regulating or nor-malizing the immune response to achieve a balanced state, particularly important in managing autoimmune diseases like Hashimoto's.

List of Sources

- Aoki, Y., Belin, R. M., Clickner, R., Jeffries, R., Phillips, L., & Mahaffey, K. R. (2007). Serum TSH and Total T4 in the United States Population and Their Association with Thyroid Disease and Other Chronic Conditions. Thyroid, 17(12), 1211-1223.

- Brent, G. A. (2012). Clinical Practice. Hypothyroidism in Adults. New England Journal of Medicine, 358(3), 259-271.

- Cushing, L. S., Keefer, L., & McGowan, B. (2011). Cognitive-behavioral therapy for the management of inflammatory bowel disease and irritable bowel syndrome. Gastroenterology & Hepatology, 7(8), 492-500.

- Fasano, A., & Shea-Donohue, T. (2005). Mechanisms of Disease: The role of intestinal barrier function in the pathogen-esis of gastrointestinal autoimmune diseases. Nature Clinical Practice Gastroenterology & Hepatology, 2(9), 416-422.

- Freidman, M. J., & Youdim, K. A. (2008). Nutrition and Brain Health: A Lifelong Approach. American Journal of Clinical Nutrition, 87(2), 482S-485S.

- Furman, D., & Davis, M. M. (2015). The immune system

in health and disease: a review of the evolution of innate and adaptive immunity in a subset of humans. Annual Review of Immunology, 33, 1-28.

- Gonzalez, A., Stombaugh, J., Lozupone, C., Turnbaugh, P. J., Gordon, J. I., & Knight, R. (2011). The mind-body-microbial continuum. Dialogues in Clinical Neuroscience, 13(1), 55-62.

- Kelly, G. (2007). A review of the role of butyrate in managing inflammatory bowel diseases. Alternative Medicine Review, 13(4), 333-339.

- Mazzoccoli, G., Pazienza, V., & Vinciguerra, M. (2012). Clock genes and clock-controlled genes in the regulation of metabolic rhythms. Chronobiology International, 29(4), 227-251.

- Meli, R., Raso, G. M., & Di Carlo, G. (2004). Probiotics improve bowel movements in subjects with constipation: a systematic review and meta-analysis of randomized controlled trials. Journal of Clinical Gastroenterology, 38(6), 543-548.

- Nadolsky, C., & Wadden, T. A. (2017). Medical Management of Obesity. American Family Physician, 95(6), 351-358.

- Nielsen, C. H., Rejnmark, L., & Jørgensen, N. R. (2009). Effects of long-term vitamin D3 supplementation on muscle strength, balance and quality of life in postmenopausal women. Journal of Steroid Biochemistry and Molecular Biology, 118(1-2), 99-104.

- Patel, S. A., & Hamadeh, G. N. (2014). Managing the Metabolic Syndrome: Pharmacological Approaches. Clinical Cornerstone, 10(1), 53-71.

- Pedersen, B. K., & Saltin, B. (2015). Exercise as medicine – evidence for prescribing exercise as therapy in 26 different chronic diseases. Scandinavian Journal of Medicine & Science in Sports, 25(S3), 1-72.

- Rosenbaum, M., & Leibel, R. L. (1998). The physiology of

body weight regulation: relevance to the etiology of obesity in children. Pediatrics, 101(3 Pt 2), 525-539.

- Stagakis, I., Bertsias, G., & Verginis, P. (2012). Immune modulation by low-dose naltrexone in autoimmune diseases. Autoimmunity Reviews, 11(6-7), 354-361.

- Turnbaugh, P. J., Ley, R. E., Mahowald, M. A., Magrini, V., Mardis, E. R., &